From the book (p. 140)

"At first you try to continue to live your life as normally as possible. As pain permeates all the nooks and crannies of your life, however, it begins to interfere with your usual routines and activities. You begin to question your ability to follow everyday routines. Self-care, chores, tasks, work, exercise, creativity, entertainment, socializing, and recreation — all become challenging, often undoable. Making plans or managing expectations becomes difficult or impossible. Dealing with your pain becomes more important than getting things done. Your life begins to look like a heap of good intentions, constantly undone by your latest pain flare-up. Your sense of 'life as usual' and 'everything is okay' evaporates, replaced by a mounting sense of loss ..."

For information, additional assessment forms, and
to learn about other offerings available from Dr. Weisser,
visit www.newoptionsinc.com

Praise for the Weisser Approach

"It is more important to know what sort of a patient has a disease than what sort of a disease the patient has" — a dictum heartily embraced by Sir William Osler, the father of modern medicine. Not only has Alan Weisser, PhD also embraced it, he has expanded upon it in his important book *New Possibilities: Unraveling the Mystery and Mastering Chronic Pain,* where he brings forth a knowledgeable, insightful, and effective approach to managing chronic pain. His insights into the critical importance of what life experiences each person brings to their chronic pain condition — and the meaning of their pain to them — sets the stage for his comprehensive, function-based approach to treatment. While much has been written about the psychological management of chronic pain, *the offerings of Dr. Weisser stand out for their sophistication, clarity, and applicability.* He teaches us that, in many cases, the pain may be unavoidable but the suffering can become optional. For patients and providers alike, this is an essential read."

Stanley A. Herring, MD
Clinical Professor, Departments of Rehabilitation Medicine, Orthopaedics and Sports Medicine and Neurological Surgery, University of Washington

---

"Dr. Weisser has been instrumental in caring for our mutual patients who suffer from chronic pain. *His unique methods have helped hundreds of our patients* learn to cope more effectively with chronic pain and live fuller and richer lives as a result. I am delighted he has chosen to author a book describing his dynamic approach so that many others may also benefit."

Virtaj Singh, MD
Seattle Spine and Sports Medicine

"*Seeing is believing.* That's all I need to say. Sharing patients with Dr. Weisser, I am convinced that by leading the patient through the complexity of their pain, he leads them to an existential recovery."

John D. Sinclair, MD
Anesthesiologist and Chronic Pain Management
Seattle, WA

"Chronic pain destroys lives. It stresses families to the breaking point. It drives friends apart. In many cases it leads to drug abuse. It destroys dreams and demolishes hope. For those wracked by chronic pain, returning to a life worth living may seem impossible and — without a guide — it may actually be. *Dr. Weisser is a guide who can be trusted.* I know, because I have seen how those under his care have benefited from what he is now sharing in this book. There is no magic bullet and there is no pill that will eliminate chronic pain. There is, however, a path to a better future — one in which pain can be managed, families can be reconstructed, and friendships can be re-established. Dr. Weisser has helped even some who had given up hope, to find their own path. I know, because I have referred many with chronic pain to Dr. Weisser, and I have seen the results. I applaud Dr. Weisser for sharing his knowledge. His office practice has benefited many; his book will benefit those in pain globally."

Lee S. Glass, MD, JD
Associate Medical Director
Department of Labor and Industries

New Possibilities

New
Possibilities

Unraveling the Mystery
and Mastering Chronic Pain

ALAN STEPHEN WEISSER, PhD

New Options, Inc.

LIBRARY OF CONGRESS CATALOGING-IN-PUBLICATION DATA
Weisser, Alan S, author
New Possibilities: Unraveling the Mystery and Mastering Chronic Pain, title
ISBN: 978-1-7378598-0-2
ISBN: 978-1-7378598-1-9 (EPUB)
Library of Congress Control Number: 2021920229
HEA036000 HEALTH & FITNESS / Pain Management
Includes index

Strategies for reclaiming your life from chronic pain by understanding the full impact of chronicity to all aspects of life.

PRODUCTION CREDITS
Editing: Jennifer Hager, Rachel Fudge, and Tandem Editing LLC
Book design and layout: BodyMind Books (bodymindbooks.com)

NEW OPTIONS, INC, PUBLISHER
4500 9th Avenue Northeast, Suite 300, Seattle, WA 98105 USA
To contact the author or order copies, write to info@newoptionsinc.com.

DISCLAIMER
Much of the content in this book is the result of mutual journeys of discovery with the author's clients, over many years. Proper informed consent was obtained and effective steps were taken to preserve client confidentiality and privacy in the examples given. All examples are provided solely to foster reader understanding, and have been modified to both retain the essence of the individual's experience and preserve complete anonymity.

To seeking the truth in the light of all that is.

Contents

Acknowledgments

When I thought about acknowledging all the people involved in the inspiration behind this book, the list was poignantly long, and the relationships lifelong and deep.

My understanding of chronic pain began with my own experience at age twelve when I broke my neck in a diving accident at a local pool, an event that damaged me not just physically, but emotionally, psychologically, and existentially. Blaming myself for my shaken confidence and sense of identity, I suffered until a turning point occurred, with my high school chemistry teacher, Mr. Grossmark. He was the first person in my life who recognized that my injury had not just damaged my body, but my self-image and ability to know who I truly was and what I was capable of. He helped me, by way of his chemistry tutoring, to regain much of what had been lost, supporting me to the point of doing well and teaching me in the process the value of really applying myself, not assuming limitations, and, more importantly, believing in myself.

This set the stage in my life for many others who followed and who added to this existential healing process: My first true love Joan, who had unflinching faith in me. Friends and professors that I met in college, and along the way at the beginning of my first career as a lawyer. Even during law school — when I spent the summers working as a shoe salesman, my manager, Mr. Grant, modeled just how successfully a person could redesign and recreate themselves despite great adversity. He had overcome many difficulties and tragedies and become highly successful in his work.

As I've gone through life witnessing the negative events that can happen to people and how they meet (or don't meet) those challenges, and through facing my own challenges, I have come to understand the true value of seeing possibilities that exist in suffering. I've learned why it is so important to start by looking at the reality of things.

Of all the people in my life who have inspired me and helped me on the path to self-discovery and growth, most importantly there is my wife, Sondra, the truest partner anyone could have in life. For her love and faith in me, for her patience and generosity that have sustained me, and her willingness to make sacrifices so that I could do what I needed to do for many, many, years, I can never thank her enough. My brother Michael, who's always been there for me unconditionally as both a brother and a friend. Also, my friend Matt Capobianco, my best friend from high school who I knew lifelong until his death several years ago. He was always there to remind me of who I really am. Thank you, man, wherever you are now. Thank you to my senseis Mr. Hara and Grandmaster Rico Guy for the faith they showed in me and the many valuable life lessons learned in my practice with them.

It seems there's always been someone to help me along the way. The years I spent in psychoanalysis working with Dr. Gerald Perlman added great depth to my understanding of myself and what was important to me. He inspired me before I started my private practice, which eventually led to the development of my chronic pain approach. When I was at odds with myself as to whether I wanted to do that and, for the first time in years, called Dr. Perlman to ask his advice, he did as any good psychoanalyst would do: he listened. He only said one thing, and it was as close as he ever got to telling me what to do: If you don't do it you'll live to regret it. Thank you Gerry. I didn't know how right you would be. And thank you to Dr. Alvin Pam, the head of psychology at Bronx psychiatric center where I did my internship and afterwards spent many years as a mentee of Dr. Pam — thank you, Al; you encouraged me to find my own way in the work I do.

I cannot offer enough thanks and gratitude to Dr. David Sinclair, Dr. Stan Herring, Dr. Lee Glass, and my friend and partner in my work in chronic pain, Judy Davis, master therapist. It was because of their support and encouragement and their providing opportunity that I was able to build and develop my approach to chronic pain, and help it flourish.

And most of all, thank you to all the patients who have trusted me to try to help them, and inspired me by their courage, commitment, and success in recovery.

~Alan Weisser

What to Expect from This Book

This book is both manual and workbook. It offers many approaches you and your providers might take to successfully address not just your pain but most, if not all, of the negative impacts it causes. Many of these strategies become available to you just by reading this book — you can begin to use them without further consultation. Other strategies might best be reinforced by coaching, counseling, or further education, support, and direction. The book outlines multiple possibilities and opportunities to restore your functioning and increase satisfaction in your life. It highlights how personal transformation can lead to less pain and more thriving.

In the three chapters that make up part 1, "A Holistic Understanding," you will be introduced to the basic concepts in the book: how profoundly and in how many ways chronic pain can impact your life, and how essential it is to take a holistic perspective if you are to find effective, sustainable ways of treating and living well with chronic pain.

Each of the part openers provides a summation of its section — its tools, takeaways, and bottom line. Part 2 and 3 provide the core of the book: thirteen chapters that cover the specific impacts of pain and the kinds of damages they can have on your physical, mental, and emotional self. Each chapter includes one or more sections titled "Recovery." The recovery sections corral the counters to the various negative impacts — approaches you can take to avoid or undo the havoc that living with chronic pain can cause. The concept of recovery — that, paradoxically, you can live with but be free from the potential damages wrought by pain — is adapted from the world of addiction and rehabilitation where, as with chronic pain, there is inherent complexity, and yet your challenge does not have to run or ruin your life.

Part 2, "The Physical Experience," covers physical harm. Each of the seven chapters in this section is devoted to one major category of physical impacts that can be caused by chronic pain. Each chapter presents a spectrum of potential problems in detail, followed by a recovery section filled with useful perspectives, strategies, and suggestions.

Part 3, "The Personal Experience," contains six chapters that range from day-to-day impacts to functional, existential, and mental health impacts. As in part 1 and part 4, the chapters in part 3 are structured to present an understanding of potential problems, damages, or challenges, followed by strategies for recovery.

Part 4, "The Treatment Experience," has just two chapters. The first focuses on all the obstacles — both external and internal — people may face in the treatment environment. The second provides practical help in how to successfully navigate that environment. It also presents tools, attitudes, and strategies for being a proactive patient. Together, these two chapters offer powerful ways to effectively get your needs met in the treatment environment and make the most of your relationships with your providers.

The concluding chapter contains in-depth stories of inspiration and community. These stories introduce you to individuals who have suffered from chronic pain, individuals who I have had the privilege of calling my clients. These are my heroes. You will hear about their challenges and the ways in which they took charge of their lives, mastered their situations, and went on to fulfill their potential in ways great and small. I hope this chapter will inspire you to explore your uniquely personal avenues for mastering your life and your pain.

This book reflects the breadth of situations I have worked with across the experiences of literally thousands of people suffering from chronic pain. There may be quite a few chapters that don't apply to your particular experience at all. So in the appendixes, you will find questionnaires that correspond to the material in parts 2, 3, and 4. By going through these questionnaires, you can quickly determine which sections are most relevant for you.

I have found that to be most helpful, we have to start with a discovery of what the negative realities of living with chronic pain are, in detail. From that point, as we move through the material in this book, we will enter into a discovery of your innate potential — physically, psychologically, emotionally, existentially, and in relationships — to transform suffering into possibility.

I hope that you will experience your journey in this book as I did: as an unfolding of awareness and understanding, and, finally, a blossoming of inspiration to experience your own potential in action and overcome the challenges pain presents.

New Possibilities

From Mystery to Mastery

A ny new and unprecedented challenge calls for extraordinary innovation. Chronic pain presents exactly this level of challenge: It
asks you to use your awareness, insight, and understanding to
address your suffering by *identifying and overcoming* obstacles to your
innate potential. Everyone has this potential. *You* have this potential.

This book draws on the many psychological approaches I have studied
and practiced over the past decades and the successes I have seen my
clients achieve. Every approach begins with your willingness to engage
in self-exploration. To learn about yourself, how you operate as a person,
how you cope, and how you go about getting your needs met. To learn
what works and what does not, especially when confronted by chronic
pain and its impacts. So I ask of you: As you read this book, be open to
everything you can learn to help yourself approach mastery — not just
of your pain but of yourself and your innate power. Your own process of
self-discovery will then continue to help you find your way forward.

A FOCUS ON UNDERSTANDING

Before I began working with chronic pain, I worked with many individuals with exceedingly difficult emotional and psychological problems.
In particular, I worked with people with chronic mental illness, both
hospitalized and outpatient. It was in this work that I began to understand the necessary focus of my efforts: I needed to focus in the main,
not on the diagnosis or disease but on who each person was and how
their life had been affected by their condition. It turned out that this was

best understood by learning what their condition meant to them, and how aware and capable they were of bringing their innate tools to bear to address their illness.

So I translated all the medical and psychological knowledge and techniques I had been taught toward that end. I learned to help my clients not by trying to rid them of a possibly incurable injury or disease but by reducing their suffering and dysfunction and helping them create a sense of mastery over their condition. By helping them become more empowered in any way possible.

For example, people with higher IQs are known to be better able to function, so I developed a technique to help hospitalized clients increase their IQs. I gave them tasks to help them practice attention, concentration, awareness, problem-solving skills, and teamwork. And it worked!

I learned I could also help my clients gain greater insight and mastery over their conditions by focusing on building human relationships with them. This meant aligning with what mattered to them and what gave their lives meaning. It meant showing respect for how they were trying to cope with their illness, no matter how dysfunctional their efforts might be. When I did this, I found people became more open to considering changes in their approach to coping, more willing to be creative and try something new to reach a richer outcome, one that returned a higher level of mastery over their lives.

Here is an example. In the hospital unit where I worked at the time, many patients had been in the hospital for many years and did not participate fully in treatment. Many staff members believed this meant these patients were lazy and resistant to treatment. When I started working with them, I reassured them that I was not trying to get them discharged from the hospital. Instead, I asked them what they valued about being in the hospital. As you might expect, they identified 24/7 professional help, medication, meals, a bed, and a safe environment as reasons they did not want to leave. They knew that if they were discharged to the streets of New York, they would be without any of these resources. I then asked them to identify what was not available to them in the hospital. They identified the lack of a private room, their own TV, privacy, and other personal freedoms.

When I offered to find an environment outside the hospital that would give them everything they wanted, they said they would work toward discharge to have that. My work then, to deliver on my promise, was to innovate and develop a wholly different approach to outpatient resources.

Once this was created, I was able to get many of these patients discharged successfully.

All my prior work with chronic mental illness prepared me to take on the challenge of helping people with chronic pain, and all that pain brings with it. I've been energized to evolve techniques and approaches that can help people recover. Once again, I've been challenged to build on what I know and identify how it applies to helping people achieve mastery over a major life challenge. All the information in this book comes from this one common focus and experience: As my clients and I fully grasp what can and has happened to them due to their injury, we respond by focusing on removing obstacles to their innate potential.

UNDERSTANDING THE IMPACT

When I began this work, I knew that incurable injuries and chronic disease often lead to persistent pain. In my initial efforts at treatment, I never ignored this reality. My evaluations focused on physical and psychological diagnosis and symptoms and on the level of impact on functioning. Over time, this exploration revealed the apparent impact of something *more* than the specific injury, disease, anxiety, or depression. As I looked at the impact on functioning, it was obvious that many more things were playing a role in my clients' pain and dysfunction.

These "many more things" seemed to be connected to my observation of people's confusion when I first began to work with them. They were confused about why the pain they reported was greater than their providers expected, and why their benefit from treatment was less than their providers expected. They also seemed unsure of what their diagnosis was, what it meant, and what to expect. They were confused about what their treatments were for, how the treatments were supposed to work, and what to expect from them. I realized that this sense of mystery and confusion was making it hard for both me and my clients to understand and manage their pain.

In seeking to unravel the mystery, I began charting what I later came to call *collateral damages*. Then I reached out to health care providers for more concise information. My clients' providers were most gracious and helpful but were also somewhat shocked to learn that their patients felt so confused. Providers also admitted to their own mystification about their patients' high pain reports and limited responses to treatment. This process became a mutual journey of demystifying chronic pain: for myself, my clients, and their providers.

Just what was affecting people's high pain ratings and poor treatment outcomes? What were the things we had not understood or considered?

At that point, I remembered one of the most compelling statements a previous client had once made to me. She said, "When I had my psychotic break, I fell out of life. And I haven't been able to get back in since." This began my search not just for what had happened to my clients because of their pain, but what it all meant to them.

The Meaning of the Mystery

Like ripples of damage and disability, chronic pain's impact is comprehensive and ever expanding. I continue to discover more beyond what I originally knew. You need to be on the lookout as well. The impacts of pain can and do multiply and change over time. Based on this understanding, I start with a person's descriptions of their injury or illness and a report of events since their injury. A client might tell me they have lost abilities, tasks, and activities, lost a job or career opportunities, or are experiencing anxiety and depression. Then I ask, "What do these events mean to you?"

For example, losing a job might be extremely important to one person, but not so much to another. When I wanted to understand how collateral damage affects someone, how it might be impacting them, I needed to know the meaning of that event to that specific person. Each time I used this approach with a client, it began to explain their mysterious pain ratings and limited response to treatment.

For example, when I met Sarah, an accomplished orthopedist, she had developed a significant spinal injury that first threatened to undermine her career and eventually caused her to be unable to work. For years she had been dedicated to her job to the extreme. She had attached her value as a person to her ability to excel and achieve at a remarkably high level in all aspects of her life. Then her pain had undermined her ability to function this way.

She felt challenged in her sense of identity, purpose, and meaning. This made her feel, in her words, "worthless." She believed she was "weak" to be so strongly affected by her pain. She blamed herself for her inability to make more progress and saw herself as a "failure" for not being able to master the pain. She began to experience significant levels of depression, anxiety, and anger, but she felt ashamed of these reactions, experiencing them as further signs of her deficiencies as a person. However, neither Sarah nor her providers had discussed or considered the *meaning* she attributed to her experiences with her pain. All were unaware that the way she thought about her pain could both add to it and interfere with her rehabilitation.

Sarah's mental state had caused her to be unwilling to consistently engage in her prescribed physical therapy, home exercises, acupuncture, and massage. She attributed her difficulties in following her treatment plan and making progress to some shortcoming on her part. This thinking undermined the physical and functional benefit of these interventions. She was also resistant to dealing with the emotional impact of her pain, and until she engaged in counseling, this added to her anxiety and depression. No one, including Sarah, was taking her existential issues into account, and this also undermined her faith in treatment and in her providers — limiting their ability to help her.

At the time I met her, Sarah's depression was worsening to a dangerous level. But once we discussed what her pain and its impacts meant to her, things changed. We could see how her approach to coping was compounding her problems. We explored all the different ways she might preserve her self-worth that didn't depend on her ability to excel. What if her approach to self-worth could become more grounded in her desire, her intention, and her perseverance to do well — whether she "succeeded" or not?

We also discussed Sarah's tendency to judge herself and how it was disempowering and interfering with recovery. We worked on ways she could *value* her negative emotions and sense of vulnerability, and not see them as weakness. This led to exploring different approaches to coping and alternate ways to lessen the impact of her injury and her emotional suffering. As a result of this counseling work, Sarah became more committed to her treatment and rehabilitation. She became less depressed and anxious. She was much more willing to work with her providers.

Sarah made significant progress in rehabilitating her physical and emotional pain, and she eventually preserved both her career and her performance standards. She became better able to cope with all challenges in her life and had a stronger sense of herself — based not on her performance but on her value as a whole person.

Many chapters in this book explore the variety of impacts that can occur post-injury: physical, day-to-day, situational, functional, and experiential. There are many more collateral damages than you might expect, and this number is multiplied when you take each person's uniqueness into consideration. They cover many aspects of life that most people do not consider. Together, these impacts add up to an existential crisis. *Chronic pain damages meaning.*

An Existential Treatment Model

Once I understood the significance of collateral damages to the individual, I began to change my treatment model. The standardized psychological approaches to pain management, such as cognitive-behavioral therapy, are not enough to address an existential crisis. For an existential crisis, an existential, meaning-based response is also needed. Along with the traditional psychological approaches based on practical, behavioral, and cognitive change models, this combined approach is reflected throughout this book.

> "For an existential crisis, an existential, meaning-based response is needed."

Understanding the mystery in chronic pain means knowing it is not just about a physical injury but about a damaged life. This clearly suggested to me that it would take more than management to help someone thrive. That I should seek ways to help my clients master their pain, to marginalize and minimize the control that pain can have. But how would I accomplish this?

From Mystery to Inspiration

I've always been driven by a desire to explore the limits of what is possible, to take on challenges that seem almost too much to overcome. This was true, for example, of an injury I sustained at a young age, which led to my lifelong study of the martial arts.

I first became aware of martial arts when I was a child, by watching Saturday-afternoon kung fu movies. The dubbing was laughable, the stories often incomprehensible, but the kung fu moves were artful in form and application. More importantly to me, the stories often involved the hero facing great personal and physical challenges. These included the process of mastering the art, which often meant dealing with serious injuries and limitations and great emotional challenges. The heroes accomplished all of this through determination, perseverance, inspiration, help from their teachers and fellow students, and nonacceptance of their limitations. Everything they worked to overcome led to personal growth, evolution, and— eventually — mastery. I felt a keen interest in and affinity with this process.

Then, at age twelve, I broke my neck in a diving accident at a local swimming pool. I survived. I was not paralyzed. But I was told by my doctors that I could not engage in sports for the rest of my life. I was too "fragile."

I unwillingly abided by their advice until I went to college. My accident had caused me to lose my sense of worth and my identity as an adventurous, risk-taking individual. But I was looking for a way to get back as much as I could. I was intrigued by the idea that there must be something out there that could help me overcome my physical limitations and the emotional and psychological harm I had suffered from my injury.

So, during college — against advice, and perhaps against better judgment — I decided to give martial arts a try. Perhaps I could be like one of the heroes in a kung fu movie! Perhaps I could master all my challenges — physical, emotional, psychological, and existential.

In martial arts, the underlying principle is that you do not know your limits unless you push them — with physical safety at the center. Given my desire to recapture an important part of my life, I was highly motivated to try. It turned out that I could do more than I'd been told I could — and more than *I* thought I could.

To participate in martial arts, I had to change many of the patterns in how I operated as a person. I had to show respect for my fear and other feelings. I had to acknowledge my limits and let others help me. I had to acknowledge *all* the impacts of my injury and how they had affected me. Most importantly, I had to challenge myself to find out who I really was and what I was capable of.

I learned something from this that has shaped my entire life in a positive way. I really did not know my true self or the scope of my potential. In exploring this, I became inspired to find ways to overcome the challenges life had presented me with. Like the heroes in the movies, I faced many obstacles along the way — and still do — but martial arts have now set the tone for how I approach anything that seems impossible to overcome.

I practice martial arts to this day. My neck has never been a limiting factor or problem. This practice continues to be central to my personal growth and my sense of unlimited potential.

For me, being involved with people who are trying to preserve what life of theirs they can, to recover their losses, and to get back to lives they value is familiar and personal. Just as I helped myself, I became inspired to find ways to help others. I realized that if people can connect to the idea of changing themselves, of seeking empowerment in pushing their limits, something that had seemed impossible could happen: recovery.

Pushing limits is just another way of saying, "Let's find out what's possible." As I worked with my clients to do this, I began to understand the extent and complexity of the barriers and obstacles. For instance, a person's way of getting their needs met might help their progress — or hinder it.

The recovery sections you will find throughout this book will help you address who you are, where your barriers interfere, and how to push your limits — by tapping into what inspires you. This quest is the foundation and driving force for everything in this book.

> "Anything that helps to empower you, anything that unleashes your potential as a human being, can ultimately aid you in mastering chronic pain."

The heart of managing chronic pain is not just traditional treatments, and not just the tools that are covered in this book. It is the understanding that anything that helps to empower you, anything that unleashes your potential as a human being, can ultimately aid you in mastering chronic pain. You do not have to be dependent on health care providers and practitioners. You do not have to be dependent on the approaches recommended in this book. Tapping into what inspires you, tapping into what matters to you, will lead to your innate potential to overcome whatever you are dealing with.

Communal Purpose

From my martial arts classes, I also gained a sense of alignment of purpose with my senseis and fellow students. We were all inspired by the challenges of training to reach our potential. The partnership of teacher and students is considered the highest form of martial arts mastery. Similarly, all my experiences, both personally and with clients, underscore the critical importance of community and emotional connection with others in the recovery process.

Great power is available when inspiration flows not just from within you but from others as well — and from one person to another. I have witnessed this firsthand with my clients. My deep conviction that there is hope in challenging the limits of what is possible, joined with my clients' growing understanding of what inspires them, enhances their recovery considerably.

As part of my chronic pain practice, I include a client's spouse or significant other in some of our sessions. People close to someone with chronic pain often suffer at a significant emotional and psychological level as well — in part because successful communication and understanding in trying to help their loved one is hard to achieve. Sometimes just trying to understand creates friction and emotional disconnection. Partners and family members often do not feel they can be a part of their loved one's recovery, nor can they relieve their own stress from it.

To address this, I work to educate my clients' loved ones about collateral damages and how they affect pain and recovery. We work on the most helpful orientation and approach to feeling more empowered and more effective in helping. This also involves helping them deal with their own suffering and understanding their role in the recovery process. We work together to find a pathway to unite their loved one's striving toward inspiration with their own desire to help. They become part of the team — a partner and an ally, not just a helpless, unhappy onlooker. By coming to terms with their own challenges, they are helping not only their significant other but also themselves master the impact of chronic pain.

Like you, your loved one can learn how to tap into their own potential to deal with the emotional, psychological, and existential suffering — yours and theirs — that is caused by your chronic pain.

Finding mutual intent and purpose, mutual inspiration, with others is a major factor in recovery. The critical importance of this has been brought home to me in several cases. One story that stands out dramatically is that of Walker, a veteran of the US Armed Forces who had served in Afghanistan.

Walker had multiple herniations in his back, and in addition to chronic pain, he also suffered from PTSD from his experiences in combat. The impact from his physical injuries prevented him from working, and produced major friction and arguments with his wife of many years. This deepened his depression and sense of helplessness. Meanwhile, the disconnect between him and his wife, Andrea, had them on the brink of a divorce. Walker did not feel understood or supported in his suffering. Andrea was frustrated with his reactions and did not know how to help him.

I met with both for several months using the process described above. Eventually, Walker no longer felt alienated and alone in his suffering, and neither did Andrea. She had gained understanding and learned skills that helped her manage her own stress more effectively. Their joint efforts succeeded in restoring their marriage and family cohesiveness.

Perhaps even more important, this process led to Walker's discovery of a true vocational passion. The exploration of space was inspiring to him, and he had always dreamed of being involved in spacecraft engineering. This realization led him to enter and succeed in an educational program that would lead toward this goal. His passion helped him overcome his pain and depression and make a successful start toward his dream his dream.

All individuals who are involved with people in chronic pain can cheer them on in their struggle. They can tap into their own inspiration to find ways to help. Inspiration within and from your community and powerful emotional connection and support are in fact two essential elements in mastering your chronic pain.

From Inspiration to Invention

The recovery sections offer not just techniques you can use but also examples of how others have used them. Because you yourself, and what you bring to the challenge, are an essential part of the continuing process of discovering meaning and inspiration.

Barbara's story offers a useful illustration of this. Barbara was living with the aftermath of multiple back injuries, which could, on occasion, cause a great deal of pain. At one point, she was having a major flare-up of pain, and nothing she had learned and mastered during our several years of work was helping. When she recognized this, she paused and thought about the things that really mattered to her. She remembered that being kind to people was important to her, and she decided to spend the rest of the day engaging in random acts of kindness. By the end of the day, she reported, she had 40 percent less pain.

> "It is your uniqueness, your unique sense of meaning that will lead you toward mastery."

Not all my clients begin their recovery inclined toward invention. However, those who come to understand this approach embrace more than techniques. They understand that they have a major role in finding a way to bring meaning back into their lives. It is your uniqueness, your own sense of purpose, your unique sense of meaning that will lead you toward mastery.

We are all reminded of our potential when we see others overcome the impossible. The mother going beyond her physical strength to lift a car to save her child. The brilliant scientist Stephen Hawking, who, unable to move or even speak without the aid of a computer, lived a long life pursuing his passion for scientific discovery. We cheer at every sports event where some player does something beyond what people have done before. We are inspired when Nelson Mandela, after years of torture and imprisonment, brings his unique strength and understanding to help unite his country. For these and many others, suffering is not the end but the beginning of understanding and expressing what you, I, and all humans really are: unlimited potential accessed through inspiration. We are designed to use this potential in the face of major challenges. But how?

Infinite Potential

How do we access our infinite potential? While the answer may seem obvious to some, to most people I believe it comes as it did with me — with potentially profound implications: We are all the ongoing products of evolution. All living things are. We are designed with evolutionary potential and the equipment to adapt to any challenge, to survive and even to thrive. What we have available — not just as individuals but as human beings — to address any challenge, including those presented by chronic pain, is our infinite potential. This conviction has guided my questions, observations, and discoveries.

In my work with people with chronic mental illness, people with conditions that had a high negative impact on their ability to function, I learned to focus on function and meaning. When I did, I was amazed at what my patients were able to do. This taught me about the powerful potential they were able to mobilize when they were, first, motivated by something that mattered to them and, second, had learned how to use their evolutionary equipment.

Then I brought this focus on function and meaning into my process of trying to help my clients with chronic pain deal with their challenges. Following my growing findings about collateral damages, I made that a focus too. What would help people produce the most optimal response to the challenge of chronic pain? How could these three areas of focus — function, meaning, and collateral damage — be applied to uncover what would help them the most?

This orientation, and similar general approaches evolving in psychology, led me to develop cognitive-existential techniques: re-constitutions, re-conceptualizations, and new approaches that had even more power to help my clients. Using these techniques revealed the different aspects of what I call an *existential immune system.* Over many years now, my work has continued to uncover ways to use the existential immune system's tools most effectively and efficiently.

In other words, your infinite potential operates through your existential immune system.

THE EXISTENTIAL IMMUNE SYSTEM

You are probably aware of your body's physical immune system. This system has many elements and processes. For example, it has white blood cells, antibodies, a complement system, a lymphatic system, a spleen, bone marrow, and a thymus. All of these elements fight threats to your body's healthy functioning. They are designed to clearly detect and defend by being diverse, specific, and, most especially, adaptive.

Evolution has also provided you with an existential immune system. It is like other immune systems in the body, but more: It is the master system. It relates to all elements of your needs. It supports all aspects of functioning: physical, emotional, psychological, and existential. It is designed to react to all challenges, no matter what their nature, and no matter what part of your functioning they affect. It is essential for responding to challenges that affect your most important needs.

Chronic pain is one of these challenges. How your existential immune system reacts to chronic pain depends on your system's current level of functionality. This depends on your awareness of this system, its tools, and its processes, and your level of competence with them. Learning to consciously use this system and its features is something like learning how to use a computer. Many of us understand the value of a computer and can execute different functions. However, learning a computer's full capabilities — and using those capabilities to accomplish specific tasks — requires a deeper level of study and assistance. The rest of this introduction will outline the elements I discovered during my initial journey of understanding and exploring the tools of the existential immune system.

Thoughts and Feelings

Thoughts and feelings are at the core of all human experience. They are critically important elements of the existential immune system. They are also the most central point of access for interventions. How we use our thoughts determines our feelings, and our feelings, in turn, generate thoughts. Thoughts and feelings are the ultimate manifestation of everything that happens in human awareness.

An individual's thoughts are determined by their perception of their experience, which in turn is determined by their awareness of whatever is relevant to what's happening. When I decided to work with my clients' current perceptions and level of awareness of their condition — along with what tools they could bring to bear on it — I soon realized that this focus would open the path to evolving and thriving.

I began to study the perceptual experiences and reactions manifested by my clients with chronic pain. I looked for patterns and implications. What I found reconfirmed the importance of awareness, perception, thoughts, and feelings in human behavior — something that has been known in psychology for a number of years. Whole schools of psychology have been built around the significance of these elements. Cognitive therapy emphasizes the importance of thinking. Other therapies, like rational emotive behavior therapy, psychoanalysis, and psychodynamic psychotherapy, put a great deal of value on emotions. No matter the approach, they all recognize that our lack of awareness can lead to perceptions of our own experience that are central to why we suffer — and central to positive therapeutic change.

Anxiety and Anger

Human emotions are not just psychological, physical experiences. Human emotions — all of them — are part of our existential tool set, and each one has a unique function. But which emotions are most central to the operation of the existential immune system and to dealing with the threats to needs that are so common in chronic pain?

Early on, I observed that people with chronic pain experience a great deal more anxiety and anger than even people with some of the most emotionally severe cases of non-physical pain. There are many teachings and points of view on the operation of these two emotions and on their impact and possible value. Because of my interest in evolution and function, I began to wonder if these emotions were no more than a source of suffering — or could they possibly have some *useful* functional purpose?

> "Anxiety is a warning system to alert you when your needs are being threatened."

I began to explore what was provoking these feelings in my chronic pain clients. Ultimately, this led me to the observation that anxiety and anger are always tied to a threat to important needs. As it turns out, you will never experience anxiety or anger unless your needs are being threatened.

Next, I wondered if somehow these emotions might somehow be related to helping to deal with threats to needs. I theorized that anxiety was a warning system — like a fire alarm — to alert you when your needs are being threatened. It is a master warning system for all needs, whether pain, hunger, or thirst, which relate to specific physical needs, or emotional, psychological, social, or other survival needs.

While it is critical to be made aware of threats to your needs, you also need to be able to take action to reduce or eliminate the threat. For this, you need power, focus, and energy. It turns out that this power is supplied by anger, whose function is to remove the threats to your needs — ideally by reducing or eliminating them in a constructive way.

I have tested this understanding of anger and anxiety across several thousand clients, and it has proven accurate.

Having discovered this, I wondered how there could be such misunderstanding about these emotions. Most people think of anxiety as weak and shameful, or of anger as bad and destructive. Neither of these judgments are true. Anxiety is not weakness. It is not shameful. When we experience a threat to our needs, it produces anxiety. We may feel momentarily rattled—just like when a fire alarm goes off. Nothing about this emotion is weakness, whether we react usefully or less so. Anger produces a surge of energy. Behaviors like yelling, screaming, and hitting are not anger; they are a mismanagement of a useful, necessary emotion. In other words, anxiety disorders and anger management issues are caused not by the emotions themselves but by ignorance of what anxiety and anger are designed for and how to use them effectively.

Then how were these misconceptions created? Exploration of many clients' childhoods revealed that children are not often helped to understand the purpose and use of these strong emotions. Perhaps adults did not model the constructive use and expression of their own emotions. Certainly anger and anxiety can be unpleasant, and their function is not as obvious as the function of thirst or hunger. But these two emotions are designed for incredibly important purposes, nonetheless. You will find in-depth discussions of anxiety and anger in chapter 16, "Mental Health Impacts and Risk Factors." Here I outline the concepts that underlie all the information in this book, the principles that will help you better understand and use your existential immune system.

FIVE PRINCIPLES FOR OPTIMIZATION

Over time, I built on what I knew of theories and practices that could enhance use of the existential immune system and looked to see how these practices applied in a chronic pain situation. This eventually led to identifying an effective approach to self-discovery, personal evolution, and mastery of the existential immune system. The following five principles have proven to be extraordinarily helpful in the work to optimize this system: the survival triad, evolutionary-based thinking, conflict embracement, self-regard, and a meaning-based childhood.

The Survival Triad
Understanding the purpose of anxiety and anger led me to develop cognitive-existential techniques that would optimize their use, all part of an

approach I call *the survival triad*. The concept behind it is simple: Humans have many needs. We need a warning system to let us know when our needs are threatened, and we need to be able to take action to counter the threats. Learning to use anxiety and anger effectively — rather than trying to avoid them or shut them down — makes it possible to let go of dysfunctional coping mechanisms. If you know how to use your emotions, it becomes much less likely you will ever feel overwhelmed by or suffer from them. In fact, it's much more likely you will feel *empowered* by them.

The survival triad relates not just to the optimal use of feelings but to the use of thoughts as well. In other words, the survival triad is a tripod composed of needs, feelings, and thoughts. Specifically, understanding how to use your feelings and thoughts to protect your needs. When you operationalize the use of anxiety and anger, you can make the best use of your thoughts, knowledge, and wisdom.

When I am teaching clients this technique, we first determine the thoughts that suggest a threat to needs. Next, we rate the threat for its existential importance and the level of anxiety produced. We then use the motivational power of anger to identify the cognitive processes, thoughts, knowledge, and wisdom that can reduce or eliminate the threat. If doing so results in diminishing anxiety, we know we have identified the right threat and the optimal solutions. This underscores the second most important function of anxiety: It is a monitoring system for finding the optimal solutions to threats. This is the origin of the expression "Trust your gut."

Of course, the survival triad also helps you use the best, most useful forms of thinking.

Evolutionary-Based Thinking

Thoughts are how we articulate and understand experience. So which forms of thought are the most important for successful operation of the existential immune system? This relates to the second principle: To make best use of your thoughts, you need to differentiate between the types of thinking that support functioning and the types of thinking that are not helpful. Once these are determined, there are well-developed cognitive techniques to neutralize or eliminate the thoughts that do not help.

Unhelpful forms of thought include judgmental thinking, assumptions, rationalizations, ignorance-based thinking, magical thinking, and negative beliefs-based thinking. These types of thinking are neither accurate nor empowering. Why? They are all affected by distortions, inaccuracies, and incomplete information. They are damaging in many human situations, but even more so with chronic pain — yet it is in chronic pain that they are even more likely to occur, given the multiple threats to needs that arise. It is a very human tendency to simplify threats so that they can more easily be dealt with. However, no simplification will help you if it requires that you sacrifice the truth.

When I started to view thinking as a survival tool provided by human evolution, I could begin to recognize the most useful aspects of this tool. The types of thinking with the most potential to help you meet challenges are analysis, synthesis, common sense, practicality, creativity, innovation, and strategy. These are accompanied by memory, knowledge, wisdom, and awareness. All of these are best applied to reducing the threats *under the guidance of anxiety and anger.*

In-depth discussions of how to neutralize unhelpful thinking and promote helpful thinking will be found throughout this book and are concentrated in chapter 10, "Psychological Challenges," and chapter 15, "Operating-System Impacts."

Conflict Embracement

The third principle for optimizing the existential immune system is conflict. What is conflict? Why is conflict important to the existential immune system?

When people are in chronic pain, negative emotions and differences between self and others tend to run rampant. They are often more intense and more numerous the more seriously a person's needs are being threatened. Conflict in relationships between spouses, family, friends, or providers can lead to a loss of emotional support and connection and needed professional help, which, as you will see, is central to recovery.

In my clinical practice, I considered many successful approaches to conflict resolution, only to realize that the existential impact of chronic pain presents unique challenges to the effectiveness of these approaches. To overcome these challenges, I looked for the essence of what is happening in conflict from a functional perspective. What is called *conflict resolution* need not be thought of as a technique for dealing with disagreements. Instead, I look at conflict as a natural process meant to be embraced, not avoided. This understanding led me to an approach that could have more existential impact — a technique known as *conflict embracement.*

A functional understanding of conflict is that it is just a difference between people. However, people often confuse a difference that is supremely important to them with being right or having a right to impose their understanding on others. No matter how important your differences with someone may be, you can instead conceptualize them as an invitation to seek understanding and connection with each other. From a survival perspective, we humans need each other. Our differences can bring us together if we understand the mechanisms for doing that. Negative reactions to a person we are in conflict with don't have to destroy a bridge meant to keep us together; they can instead be the gateway to engaging.

> "No matter how important your differences with someone may be, you can conceptualize them as an invitation to seek understanding."

All conflict resolution techniques provide rules and structure for the process. In conflict embracement, one leads with feelings. When you have a difference with someone, the most authentic part of that experience is how that person's behavior made you feel and how that person may be feeling themselves. Those feelings — on both sides — are likely to be anxiety and anger.

We generally don't want to feel anxiety and anger toward people we care about, because these emotions break the connection to the other. But you now know much more about the uses of anxiety and anger. As you begin to embrace the conflict, being right or wrong becomes much less relevant than building the connection you want and need. Start by stating your feelings and your intention: "What you just said made me feel angry at you, and I don't want to feel that way."

I developed the techniques of *resolution communication* to successfully address interpersonal conflict. The four steps in resolution communication are permission, disclaimer, reassurance, and pitch. These steps, which are spelled out fully in chapter 18, "Mastering the Treatment Experience," have been incredibly powerful with the relationship issues created by the impacts of chronic pain. The resolution communication techniques help people with chronic pain and their providers and loved ones become more comfortable in considering their needs to be equally important. This approach can help you undo obstacles to connectivity and support relationships that are critical to recovery.

Self-Regard

Self-worth is at the core of the existential immune system, and the fourth principle — self-regard — is about making sure to consider your own needs as important as anyone else's, and to assert them whenever threatened. Self-regard means seeing your needs as equal — not just to others' needs but to different needs within yourself as well. This helps you make sure your needs are honored without internal or external dissonance.

For example, consider the need to be responsible versus the need for self-care. These needs are often at odds with each other. And given how many needs are challenged by chronic pain, conflicts between your own and others' needs can be pervasive and highly stressful. Whatever choice you make, there will likely be some compromise and emotional cost. The goal of the self-regard principle is to minimize the cost, eliminate regret or resentment, and evoke compassion for the difficulties that being human can create.

The technique for exercising self-regard involves four phases, which are discussed in more detail in chapter 18, "Mastering the Treatment Experience." These questions help you uncover what you really want or need to do once you are fully considering your own needs, the importance of the relationship in which a conflict of needs is occurring, the level of reciprocity in the relationship, and the cost of either decision. This analysis applies in any situation where there is a conflict between your internal needs, or between what you want and what somebody else wants. Only by considering and acting consciously in each situation can you be certain that you are deciding in a way you can afford and that you won't regret.

> "Only by considering and acting consciously in each situation can you be certain that you are deciding in a way you can afford and that you won't regret."

In this practice of self-regard, you may be surprised to find that you act in many of the same ways you have in the past, but now you know that you are doing so based on *your choice* and not the dictates of some aspirational values or prior conditioning. Functioning in this way, you can increasingly hope to find both self-love and the true love of others.

A Meaning-Based Childhood

To fully understand how a person operates as an adult — in their social interactions and their relationship with themselves — it is important to study the lessons they learned as a child. Experiences in childhood are critical to shaping how the existential immune system operates. Applying a meaning-based understanding of childhood reveals how a person has come to think of themselves, what they value or do not value in themselves, what they believe they are entitled to, how they resolve their differences, and what shape their thinking and feeling takes.

The existential immune system provides each person with the raw materials for developing amazing tools and capacities. These raw materials are engaged at conception, through gestation, through birth, and throughout childhood. However, many internal and external factors influence how our systems are shaped and nurtured, and whether they develop fully so that we can operate in a healthy way.

Much of this process occurs as an individual grows from infancy through childhood and through the various stages of development of feeling and thinking. As humans, we learn not just by what we experience but by what it comes to mean to us. Given any child's limited awareness, the meaning we attribute to our experience is often based on data that is not what it seems. This can lead to the development of beliefs and modes of operation that create obstacles to the healthy use of the full existential immune system.

To change this, it is important both to sort out what non-user-friendly lessons were learned and to use the other four principles to modify and upgrade one's existential operating system in the here and now. Solutions are packed throughout the book but particularly in chapter 10, "Psychological Challenges," chapter 15, "Operating-System Impacts," and chapter 16, "Mental Health Impacts and Risk Factors."

Together, these five principles — the survival triad, evolutionary-based thinking, conflict embracement, self-regard, and a meaning-based childhood — can break through most obstacles to optimal operation of the existential immune system. They were developed specifically to respond to the unique challenges of chronic pain but apply to any threat to optimal human functioning. They are the product of exploring functioning and meaning and combining cognitive approaches with structural techniques and concepts of existential connectivity. These five principles have turned out to be quite powerful in helping people develop mastery over their pain.

A QUESTION OF CHOICE

The key to tapping into potential and optimal use of the existential immune system is a willingness to engage in self-discovery, choice, and personal transformation. The path opens with an understanding of what really matters to you and what truly inspires you. The process of self-discovery I use with clients begins with an exploration of how they currently operate and how their approach to managing their lives can make better use of their evolutionary equipment. The first step in this process is to understand that how you operate as a person, in every regard, begins with choice.

Much of my approach toward self-discovery revolves around the theories and principles of existential psychology developed by psychologist and Holocaust survivor Viktor E. Frankl. In his book *Man's Search for Meaning*, Dr. Frankl shares this story:

> *We who lived in concentration camps can remember the men who walked through the huts comforting others, giving away their last piece of bread. They may have been few in number, but they offer sufficient proof that everything can be taken from a man but one thing: the last of the human freedoms— to choose one's attitude in any given set of circumstances, to choose one's own way.* (Beacon Press, 1992, page 75)

Frankl believes that self-fulfillment and a sense of purpose in one's own life are byproducts of attempting to fulfill a larger meaning, and that this is accomplished by the choices you make.

Pain does not inhibit potential. Your vast, unique potential is not limited by your pain, your personal tragedies, or your losses. However, how you choose to deal with those tragedies and losses can interfere with your ability to access your potential.

TREATING MEANING

All that you have read so far establishes a twofold path of recovery: Medical treatments of physical problems must go hand in hand with treatment for damaged meaning in your life. How can you optimize your human right to make choices that will help you master your pain? Through your own effort to *treat meaning*.

Although this may seem counterintuitive, the first step is to widen your awareness so you can see and acknowledge the negative realities of the totality of your pain experience. Treat yourself, your providers, and any others who are active in your life with a deep understanding of what has happened to you.

Acknowledging those negative realities may be terribly difficult. Even if you know where to look for this information, you may not want to see it. The extent of your losses and the threats to everything that matters to you may feel too overwhelming to approach. You may feel that acknowledging these is admitting defeat. You may prefer to stay busy or distracted, to limit awareness by limiting activity. You may try to escape through sleeping or substance abuse. You may try wishing your problems away or stuffing down any negative feelings about what has happened. You may try to avoid the truth by engaging in negative self-talk, complaining, blaming others, or pushing them away. Like many of my clients, you may have already used many of these approaches and found that they have limited long-term value.

But there are approaches that can offer sustainable benefit. When you have gained a clear awareness of your entire negative reality, you will find several alternatives in front of you that will move you forward.

You will need your ability to be completely truthful with yourself in terms of how you operate to get your needs met, and how willing you are to be true to who you are. You will need to develop a group of critical techniques and strategies to engage in constructive emotion management; embrace your vulnerability and make positive use of it; seek empowering dependence upon others, including proactive efforts to enlist help and support; and learn to value yourself unconditionally, ranking your intention and efforts over the actual outcomes. You will need to take charge of your sense of purpose and inspiration.

These strategies are the core of successfully mastering chronic pain. They require self-reflection, self-development, and conscious evolution of your current operating system. But remember this: We all have the potential to develop mastery.

The second step in treating meaning requires you to develop an even wider awareness. It asks you to become willing to be completely open and truthful with yourself about yourself. Chronic pain tends to bring to the surface any aspects of yourself that are working against you. These may be aspects of your personality, your way of coping, or the way you manage your thoughts, your feelings, or your needs. You may even find that something in your sense of identity can be a barrier. Be brave. Be persistent. There is always a way forward — as John's story shows.

John was an extraordinarily successful, hard-driving businessman and CEO of a major corporation. He was used to being in command and feeling in control of all aspects of his life, at work and at home. He was a self-described type-A personality and proud of it. He micromanaged his affairs, was reluctant to delegate to others, and believed in the saying "If you want things done right, do it yourself." In both his personal and professional life, it was his way or the highway.

This approach to life, at least by his account, seemed to have served well enough until he suffered serious injuries in a motor vehicle accident. The injuries led to a significant loss of function, threats to most of his needs, and increasing dependence on others — all situations that he hated.

He undermined the efforts of his providers with his arrogance and condescending behavior. He rejected support from friends and family, denying his need for help while deflecting his anger about his condition onto them. He was not at all comfortable with being vulnerable. He saw his own feelings of anxiety and anger as being "weak." He worked hard to cover up how he was really being affected by his pain. He spent most of his energy being angry and demanding and resisted any acknowledgment of his own needs.

These aspects of how he operated as a person were perpetuating the functional impact of his pain and preventing him from being able to master it.

John's specific constellation of personal approaches is an example of how a person may operate in a way that does not serve them well when facing chronic pain.

When I met John, my first challenge was helping him to acknowledge the negative realities of his situation. Having done that, I helped him look objectively at how he was operating as a person and how those tendencies had aided his recovery — as well as how they did not. It took time and trust for John to own the truth about himself. He found the process painful and anxiety-producing. Yet over time, he began to understand that his way of coping, his way of operating, was interfering with his ability to master his pain.

> "Mastering chronic pain is about mastering your understanding of your own experience."

Over the months that we worked on addressing this, John was eventually able to see how, despite his strengths and success, he needed to evolve in how he operated across many aspects of his personality. Acknowledging the truth about himself through self-discovery led to personal growth and a great ability to tap into all aspects of his potential. He began to achieve mastery over his pain, and this eventually led to an almost full recovery.

To this day John still feels chronic pain, but it no longer runs his life. He found new ways to value himself, even though he is operating quite differently as a person. He became comfortable with feeling vulnerable and respecting his feelings. He also became open to accepting help from others. In owning the truth about himself, he covered much of what had been lost in his life. His transformation also had the effect of enriching his relationships.

Most of my clients have, like John, found that exploring the truth about themselves is the beginning of the journey through self-discovery. The first steps can be difficult, painful, and cause a great deal of anxiety. But there is great power in this journey, because you will continually unearth and observe things about yourself that present new opportunities.

Your journey may reveal important internal influences that in the past have overwhelmed you. At times you may not be pleased with what you find. Because of this, self-discovery asks for personal courage and positive regard for yourself and your needs. But accepting what you see opens your chances to transform unhelpful patterns of thinking, feeling, behaving, and perceiving.

You will deepen your understanding of how your pain has challenged you. You will explore your potential and how to fully utilize it. You will become aware of obstacles and barriers within yourself, and you will open to evolving to overcome them. Mastering chronic pain is about mastering your understanding of your own experience, what matters to you, who and what you really are, and most importantly, accessing your potential.

Every individual is different. Each person has their own configuration of ways they operate in the world and get their needs met. Over the course of several thousand clients, I may have seen just as many ways to evoke potential or interfere with it. The stories of discovery and personal evolution I share in this book can help you understand the evolutionary equipment you came into this world with, and how you yourself can use it to move from chronic pain to persistent mastery.

Tools and Takeaways for Part 1

Treating the total you is essential to mastery and is the core of success for clients who reclaim their lives from pain.

Four questionnaires that pertain to part 1 can be found in appendix A:

- Physical Impacts Inventory
- Post-Injury Physical Experience Inventory
- Emotional and Psychological Impacts Inventory
- Physical Impacts Checklist

The thought and attention you take in filling out these self-assessment tools will begin your education about the hidden pieces of your pain experience.

Bottom Line

It is critical to understand the full scope of chronic pain's impact on your life and who you are as a person. This is the crucial missing piece in successful treatment.

PART 1

A Holistic Understanding

Chapter 1

Lost in Translation

People don't always appreciate how life-altering chronic pain can be. This is true of both patients and their health care providers. But if you're reading this book, it's likely you have experienced the impact of pain and are tired of feeling helpless to understand, manage, or successfully communicate about your pain and the way it has affected your life.

Chronic pain offers a challenge to the very possibility of a full or satisfying life. And yet a diminished life need *not* be the inevitable outcome. Chronic pain can actually lead to a life of transformation and a state of thriving. Sound unbelievable?

In my practice as a clinical psychologist, I specialize in helping people recover from chronic pain. I have learned, from thousands of clients, what gets lost in the translation from the experience of pain to the response to it, and how to help people shift from chronic suffering and dysfunction in life to recovery of both function and emotional satisfaction. I understand how you can empower yourself to shift from coping to thriving, and I wrote this book to share what I've learned.

HOW THE STORY STARTS

Michelle is an accountant and a lifelong athlete who developed chronic, disabling shoulder pain. Initially, this pain did not directly affect her ability to do her job — but the time off required for treatments did. Over time, her injury failed to respond to treatment, despite Michelle seeing several specialists and undergoing several different tests and approaches to treatment, all promising to help.

For several months before I met her, Michelle had worked a reduced schedule. At work and in her personal life, the pain began to undermine her performance and her ability to participate. The pain, and the stress it caused, was also beginning to overwhelm her emotionally. A younger colleague received a promotion that Michelle had hoped for, and she could feel her career trajectory slipping away. Her pain was now challenging her social relationships and all her valued tasks and activities: She had always been a competitive athlete but could no longer do any athletic training. Her friends seemed to be deserting her, and there was a possibility her fiancé would call off their wedding plans. She was feeling abandoned by her providers.

Her primary care physician referred Michelle to me as a last-ditch effort to "get to the bottom" of her pain.

"I think he believes the pain is all in my head," Michelle told me once she'd settled in. "He says there's no reason why I should still be having so much pain. Both my surgeon and physical therapist have given up on me, and I think my doctor is next. And maybe he should. I don't think anybody can help me. I'm going to have to live with this pain for the rest of my life."

Like many people with chronic pain who arrive at my psychology practice, Michelle was frightened, confused, cynical, and disheartened. She feared that more time would be wasted, with yet another doctor, in a fruitless search for the "magic cure" for her suffering. When she came through my office door, reluctantly, she believed that seeing me meant she had run out of "real" treatment options.

Despite all of this, Michelle was desperate for hope. She believed that the treatment she had received from her medical providers — however expert, thoughtful, and well-intended — had somehow fallen short. Knowing she had only a limited understanding of her condition and treatments, Michelle felt that her providers had not been able to explain why the treatments had failed. She wondered if her diagnosis was adequate to address and treat her injury.

With all these burgeoning doubts, her trust in her providers had eroded. Also, she had not experienced any clear handoff from one provider to another, so her treatment didn't seem well organized or coordinated. Instead, it felt fragmented and confusing. She wondered, as many patients do, "Who is in charge of my treatment? Do my providers talk to each other? Why do they often seem at odds with one another?"

When people like Michelle receive expert and state-of-the-art diagnosis and treatment that fails to meet expectations, they often feel that the whole situation is unfair. They're suffering but can't get to the truth of their condition — or understand how to get better. Despite their providers' best efforts and intentions, they often feel ignorant about their actual medical situations. They feel abandoned and increasingly helpless to reverse the downward spiral created by their pain. Their treatment experience has failed to help them understand their pain, come to terms with it, or learn how to minimize its impact in their lives.

This leads to people feeling powerless to manage their pain. What's worse, those suffering from chronic pain often feel that their lack of success — in all their efforts to find a remedy — is a *personal* failure. Why does this happen?

A SYSTEM OF HARM

Injuries that cannot be directly or easily cured lead to chronic physical pain. Once this occurs, you have two problems: the initial injury, and what happens to you because the pain doesn't end. It is not just the continuation of pain but the combination of the pain *and* its disabling collateral damages that makes chronic pain a life-altering natural disaster. Once this happens, the actual pain from the initial injury is distorted and magnified. It becomes more difficult to understand and more harmful. When pain damages your physical, psychological, emotional and existential life, it becomes a system of harm.

Chronic pain cannot be understood and treated optimally without an understanding of the entire system of harm. To succeed, you and your providers must know not just what happened to your body but what has happened to your life because of your injury — and exactly what it means to you. When this doesn't happen, people like Michelle — late in the game, after a long, painful, life-crushing search for answers — arrive at my door, without the knowledge they need, fearing I will tell them they're crazy.

THE CONFUSION IN CHRONIC PAIN

Modern diagnostics can measure a million things — but not pain! Pain comes with a sense of mystery. It is a subjective experience. Your pain cannot be directly measured, felt, or observed by anyone else.

Many different things contribute to pain, such as the type of injury, the time in your life that it happens, and the significance it all holds in your day-to-day experience and functioning. You can say, "It hurts." You can use descriptive words like *sharp*, *achy*, *burning*, or *throbbing* to describe it. You can use the 0 to 10 pain scale to give it a rating. However, these efforts have only limited value.

For example, say you tell your doctor your pain is an 8, on a 0 to 10 scale. Your doctor says, "According to your MRI, it looks like it should be more like a 4." Then you may suspect that your doctor doesn't know what's wrong with you, while your doctor may believe you're exaggerating. Inadvertently, providers will fail to take all the variables into account — in part because they can't feel what's going on in your body, in part because they are unaware of how collateral damages are contributing to it.

People with chronic pain don't exaggerate their conditions. Providers don't intend to frighten and confuse their patients. They both end up in this state of confusion because the bulk of the realities created by chronic pain are not included in their frame of reference.

Furthermore, different providers often have different theories and conflicting ideas about how much pain they expect you to have, what is causing it, or what will heal it, and they may use very different terminology to discuss the issues. To the patient with chronic pain, it's like the Tower of Babel. Providers' different interpretations of the problem can create confusion about both the understanding and the treatment of chronic pain and may not end up working toward a unified purpose or collective success. Joint efforts between providers and patients, and between one provider and another, will fail unnecessarily. When such a failure occurs, providers feel frustrated and limited in their ability to help; patients are left feeling increasingly confused and helpless.

Compounding this confusion, when people first enter treatment for chronic pain, they may assume that their various health care providers have the same idea about what causes pain and suffering, the same way of talking about it, and the same approach for helping them. Providers tend to believe this as well.

For example, specialists in chronic pain typically work with a common understanding that pain is caused by a *physical injury* or a physical system or process, and that this needs to be the focus for solutions.

However, interpretations of this physical approach can be quite different from one specialist to another, creating further confusion. In addition, by the time pain becomes chronic, the experience of pain may derive from a whole constellation of physical problems added to the original injury. In other words, your experience of pain may result from multiple types of damage in your life, many of which are not strictly "physical."

If you experience an ongoing lack of reassurance that your condition can be understood and healed, you're also likely to experience higher levels of fear. This fear adds to your pain's negative impact and sometimes creates a sense of crisis.

A HOLISTIC APPROACH

Before I became a practicing psychologist, I worked as a psychology intern in a specialized hospital training ward that treated people with chronic mental illness such as psychosis. The outcomes we achieved for patients in our hospital unit were far superior to those seen in the hospital in general. Why?

In that experience, which was my first real encounter with a holistic approach, I observed that a common language and training were utilized — a very different approach from the disjointed one described in the previous section.

Treatment plans in this hospital ward required a team approach. The team included therapy aides for day-to-day care, medical doctors, psychiatrists, nurses, case managers, psychologists, rehabilitation staff, social workers, and housekeeping staff.

In order to avoid confusion and provide coordinated care, we were all trained to treat and discuss patients based on the same question: What impact did their illness have on their ability to *function*?

These people's entire lives had been impacted by their condition. The team understood that, and we knew that regardless of our role, discipline, or specialty, we could all help each patient improve their ability to function. While mental illness was the trigger for the patient's problems, what had to be understood and treated was this bigger picture.

As professionals, as health care providers, we could counter the negative impacts of each illness in varying and unique ways. But only if we all had the same idea about the source of the patient's problem — and the same idea about how to help.

A holistic approach requires an understanding of all parts of an issue, how they are interconnected, and how they all contribute to the whole.

In that hospital ward, our common framework of language allowed us to communicate from our expertise and to effectively discuss our ideas and treatments with patients and among staff, which enabled a coordinated, integrated, and holistic understanding. We could see how each of us were helping, how each effort supported the other, and how the combination of efforts was greater than the sum of its parts.

It's similar with chronic pain. The critical thing that's missing in pain assessment and treatment today is a *holistic perspective*, one that takes into account how chronic pain is affecting your whole self and your whole life. People who don't know that may engage in a never-ending search for individual practitioners who can understand and address their needs. Yet non-holistic physical approaches are inadequate to address chronic pain, and indeed are the crux of the problem. Rather than resolving problems, they often create ever more uncertainty and confusion.

> "What's missing in treatment today is a holistic perspective, one that takes into account how chronic pain is affecting your whole self and your whole life."

For chronic pain to be successfully treated, you, your providers, and everyone involved in your care need to have the same idea about what's involved in your pain. You need the same way of discussing it and a similar holistic approach. This is an absolute necessity. Just as with chronic mental illness, successful diagnosis and treatment of chronic pain requires a shared multidisciplinary approach.

This book offers a considerable — and, honestly, possibly overwhelming — amount of information about all the different ways that chronic pain can affect someone. A holistic approach acknowledges all the impacts of chronic pain, addresses them in your treatment plan, and helps give your providers a common language and context for treating you.

When you are willing to explore the realities of your chronic pain, you will learn, as I did, how to better understand your condition and what you have the power to do about it. You will figure out what you can do, what needs to be attended to by your health care providers, and how to work more successfully together. You'll grasp the "big picture" about what has happened to you and discover the potential you have within yourself to transform your suffering into thriving.

Chapter 2

The Third Evolution

Let's take a look at the conceptual model typically used in the medical community to view chronic pain. This is a model that attributes pain only to *biological* conditions, such as viral infection, genetic expression, physical disease, or injury. This biological framework doesn't, to any important extent, make room for the *non-biological* impacts on your life caused by pain.

Chronic pain is not that simple. It is multifaceted and it evolves. Over time, it also changes the person experiencing it — in a kind of tandem evolution where both pain and person change, and each influences the other. Interestingly, your reaction to this can be yet a third kind of evolution, a personal evolution of self-discovery, increasing awareness, self-advocacy, and, most importantly, an understanding of your innate evolutionary-based potential to meet the challenges that life presents. This evolution is the key to meaningful recovery.

This chapter begins to explore the nonbiological impacts of pain on your life, and the personal resources that will help you recover.

COLLATERAL DAMAGES

Chronic pain doesn't just hurt your body. It can damage your daily ability to function — physically and otherwise — and interfere with many of your fundamental needs. Damage to those fundamental needs can be more disabling than any physical damage.

As humans we have many needs. Some basic and purely physical needs — for example, food, shelter, water, and sleep — are what allow us to survive and support overall functioning. We also have many emotional and psychological needs — for example, the need for love, affection, connection to others — and existential needs, including having a sense of purpose and meaning in life. Some needs are connected to time and place, culture, values, and circumstances; many are unique to who you are as a person. For example, someone may have a need for success, praise, or a smartphone.

"All collateral damages need to be identified as early as possible."

Pain, then, is not only physical; it can affect any if not all of your needs. It causes damage to you *as a person*. In the coming chapters, we'll see how these damages or threats to your needs can affect how much pain you experience, how often you feel it, and how it undermines your ability to function.

These damages to needs are referred to as *collateral damages*. Any collateral damage can increase your pain, and/or limit the benefits of your pain treatments or even keep them from working at all. To avoid this, all collateral damages need to be identified as early as possible. It's important to understand how they contribute to your response to treatment or exacerbate your pain, and then treat them directly, along with any physical injury.

Here are some examples of the realities — the collateral damages — that are left out of the medical/biological frame of reference:

- Changes in relationships
- Losses
- Changes in routines, activities
- Disturbances in self-identity, self-image
- Disruptions to life meaning and purpose
- Role disruption at home, at work, and in social circles
- Financial hardship or ruin
- Exacerbations to preexisting challenges
- Negative physical alterations

When these damages go unrecognized and unresolved, patients and providers are more likely to experience a failed recovery.

An existential holistic approach includes an effort to understand and address all the physical consequences of your injury *and* all of the experiential, emotional, psychological, and life impacts — as well as how they combine to cause all of the pain and suffering you experience.

This holistic model not only understands how all the impacts on your functioning from the physical injury contribute to your pain and suffering but also guides us in how to successfully treat all of the impacts, physical and otherwise. It is an approach that begins with your injury and includes all of your experiences since you were injured as well.

WHERE CHRONIC PAIN BEGINS

Pain begins with some injury or illness. When an injury becomes persistent and resistant to cure, despite medications and treatment, for longer than twelve weeks, it is called chronic. And while it is usually the obvious source of your pain and understandably the first diagnostic and treatment focus, it's only the beginning of the story of what can lead to it becoming persistent. For there is often a complexity to what contributes to your physical pain and its persistence. What can add to this is the effect on your physical, emotional, psychological, and existential state, including your social and work life, and your overall ability to function. Pain is a biological event, but it is also an event that can affect you in many ways as a person. Its damage also has *meaning*. For example, consider the difference between your reaction to a stubbed toe versus your reaction to a broken back. A stubbed toe is a momentary pain, without significant consequences. A broken back is quite serious in its potential consequences. It can change your life. Your reaction will differ in scale based not just on the amount of pain but on the impact to your life and any associated fears of that impact.

I outline a multidimensional model of pain that includes not only the initial injury or illness but also how the impacts from that injury affect you across the entire time in which you continue to have pain. It is an approach that recognizes that you are a unique individual and *pain is personal.* For example: Two individuals, one a professional lute player, break a finger. To the lute player, a great deal of personal artistic value and potential commercial livelihood is jeopardized by breaking that finger. To the non-professional, that aspect is not an aspect of their pain. Individuality is in fact very important to understanding chronic pain and different people's response to treatment.

Once pain has become chronic, the injury is in your life, not just in your body. Chronic pain causes chronic suffering—and it's important to recognize that these are inseparable. The implication is that to understand the generators of pain, and then treat them, you must look past the structural issues, past the medically defined injury, past the medical procedures and their outcomes. While these are very important, dealing successfully with chronic pain requires understanding the rest of the story. The focus needs to be on understanding your pain by understanding yourself.

If you are suffering from chronic pain, you're obviously looking for ways to reduce your pain. My challenge to you is to focus less exclusively on being helped by (and being dependent upon) medical treatment, and to focus more on understanding and using your own potential to reduce pain and restore your own functioning. To learn all you can do to restore yourself. This learning usually requires you to redefine and expand on what it means to be fully you — and to reinvent yourself, if necessary.

SELF-REINVENTION

When you undertake the effort to more deeply know yourself, you are likely to regain a positive and stronger sense of self and, ultimately, even evolve into a person who is more able to grow, flourish, and progress towards your goals — to thrive, despite the challenges you may face.

> "Your life, and especially your ability to function and feel whole as a person, must be the center of your treatment."

This work has great power to minimize and marginalize the impact that pain can have in your life. *The challenge is to turn chronic pain into an opportunity to restore yourself as a whole and complete person.* Your life, especially your ability to function and feel whole as a person, must be the center of treatment. Without recognizing the full extent to which chronic pain can create crises and destroy lives, we cannot expect ourselves to fully recover, or to return to a life of thriving.

FROM DISASTER TO RECOVERY

The diagnostic and treatment framework most commonly used to understand chronic pain today focuses on pursuing a cure instead of on recovery. A *cure* is usually understood to be the result of a substance, procedure, or process that stops, or cancels, a medical condition. It ends suffering. It heals. For example, aspirin is a cure for a headache, penicillin for bacterial infection, surgery for a broken bone, or a change of diet for high blood pressure. A cure is something that ends a medical condition, while *recovery* is a process that restores function. The notion of recovery is a more appropriate approach to addressing persistent conditions. Examples of recovery include an alcoholic maintaining sobriety or an amputee building a life not limited by what they lack.

In the case of chronic pain, recovery doesn't necessarily end the medical condition that caused the pain. What it does is return possession and control of your life to you, along with reducing suffering and offering the possibility of thriving.

Pain can cause a chronic sense of threat, or crisis. This often contributes a great deal to your stress and, in turn, increases anxiety and anger, which can undermine your ability to think and act in ways that promote recovery. Only a holistic approach such as the one described in this book can prevent chronic pain from causing persistent suffering and damage to your needs.

> "A cure is something that ends a medical condition. Recovery is a process of restoring function."

A *crisis* is an unstable, difficult, potentially dangerous but also crucial, critical situation. How does this relate to chronic pain? Like all human beings, you are biologically wired to have all your needs met. When significant needs are not being met, or are threatened by chronic pain, this creates a sense of crisis. Chronic pain thus causes personal instability and the threat of progressive losses.

When you know what the threats are, you can try to respond. But what if you are only dimly aware of how much damage you are experiencing, or what is causing so much of it? You and your providers may think, "This pain is from the injury; let's treat that." But my experience is that 25 to 50 percent of a person's chronic pain can be attributed to collateral damages — which are often not even being identified, let alone considered.

To put it another way, chronic pain impacts people the way a natural disaster does. Chronic pain can be as complex or devastating as a hurricane, earthquake, or volcanic eruption.

Most of us have witnessed, whether on the news or through personal experience, the devastation of a natural disaster. When disasters strike, everything changes for the people involved; these are life-altering events. To help the victims of disaster, it is critical to pay attention to their physical injuries and their need for medical care. However, we must absolutely attend to the other injuries the event has caused as well. Food, water, and housing may have been lost. Transportation and communication systems may have been severely damaged; employment undone; families and finances shattered. Ultimately, we need to understand and undo the damage done to the physical, emotional, and psychological lives of the people affected — damage caused by their many losses. If we do not, these damages will turn into ongoing crises.

Imagine our disaster scenario transposed to become an event or process that creates chronic pain. Medical providers respond like emergency workers: They respond to the most obvious and immediate needs of the person who is injured. The physical damage and the physical suffering it produces are clearly visible, and providers resonate with that suffering easily. But what happens if the providers and the person injured fail to recognize, or underestimate, the collateral damages caused by the injury? What if they cannot easily sort out what must be done to restore function? How will this person be able to recover?

> "A focus on recovery means a focus on restoring your full funcitoning as a person."

As badly as you may want your medical treatment to rid you of pain, most people with chronic pain agree that the loss of functioning is ultimately more devastating.

Most people don't think of chronic pain as a natural disaster, but in fact, the road to recovery requires us to assess and address it in the same fashion. If we don't, the consequences can be dire. This is easier to understand once you realize that in chronic pain conditions, eliminating the pain caused by an injury may not always be possible, given the medical methods currently available. This is one reason that *recovery* must be the focus of all your efforts.

A focus on recovery means a focus on restoring your full functioning as a person. This is considerably more attainable than full pain reduction. Recovery involves changing your relationship to pain by paying attention to all the collateral damages it causes and treating them. It also demands that you become more knowledgeable about and empowered to deal with the pain and damage. Recovery moves you toward developing the most effective coping techniques for you. This can require a transformation of how you operate as a person, in every area of your life.

This approach to recovery will most definitely reduce your suffering, and that, in turn, will reduce your physical pain.

Having worked with several thousand clients in my practice, I can say that this approach to recovery has consistently demonstrated strong results. Up to 15 percent of my clients end up with 40 to 60 percent less pain. The other 85 percent report that their pain is reduced by 25 to 40 percent, even with no obvious, diagnostically recordable physical changes.

All my clients have agreed, early on in their work with me, that with the recovery approach, they "don't feel the same way" about their pain.

In other words, they feel less stressed, affected, and controlled by it. They feel more empowered to deal with it, knowing that they don't have to rely solely on medical professionals to help alleviate their suffering. They discover that they can rely, more than they ever realized, on their own innate ability to heal their lives and thrive.

Honoring the Unique Individual

To fully understand the damage that chronic pain causes in your life, this cannot be said too many times: Your pain is more than just what happened physically. It is of critical importance to attend to what the damage done means to you *as a unique individual.*

For example, if you can't work, socialize, engage in intimacy with your partner, or engage in other normal activities for you, you will likely notice that it has a negative impact on you. However, to fully understand the impact, you'll need to ask yourself: "What does it mean to *me* that I can't do these things?" You'll need to understand the significance of the specific impacts upon you as a unique individual. This the most important information for the journey to recovery.

Consider what happened to Michelle in addition to her physical injury. Her pain caused injury to everything about her life that mattered to her: her work, her athletic activities, her friendships, her primary relationship. It had come to a point where the accumulating, untreated collateral damages had begun to undermine her sense of who she is. So, in addition to her pain, she was suffering multiple losses and teetering on an identity crisis. Her pain was challenging her core beliefs about what was possible in her life.

The medical approach to Michelle's pain had given her a diagnosis. This was a well-intentioned but narrow-minded approach. It treated her as if her injury were happening independent of her life. But, of course, her pain was not an event separate from her life but was causing ongoing consequences to it — consequences unique to what mattered most to her. To gain relief, Michelle needed to be at the center of the investigation of her pain. This would be critical to determining the meaning of her pain experience and to understanding what would help.

Looking at the Big Picture

I know that the misery experienced by people like Michelle is both heartbreaking and unnecessary. Doing something to erase that misery has become the core of my practice. Because once you get the big picture of what is happening in chronic pain, everything changes.

With Michelle, this began with a comprehensive review of her injury, diagnosis, and treatment history. Then we embarked on an extensive investigation of the collateral damage her pain had caused her.

We began this investigation with the multifaceted intake packet I developed over twenty years of taking clients' reports of the impacts of their chronic pain. It is designed to pinpoint the exact areas and the extent of the damage that pain has caused, as well as include the meaning people have made of their experiences. As Michelle worked at filling this out, I gradually learned about the big picture. Simultaneously, Michelle was introduced to a new conceptual model and a means to understand the full extent of her problem — a way to make it comprehensible.

In my first meeting with Michelle, we reviewed the intake forms, and I interpreted the findings for her. I told her, "You cannot understand what generates your pain, why treatment works or doesn't, or what your optimal treatment plan is without a clear understanding of all the ways in which the pain has damaged your life."

Filling out the forms had already begun her education about the hidden contributors to her pain problem.

Michelle then received my interpretation of the information as a validation of her suffering, not her personal shortcomings. She cried. It was obvious to her that her pain reflected so much more than just her original injury.

In addition, this conceptual grasp of her injury and the specifics of the damages she had suffered offered a possible explanation for why her pain had been such a mystery to her and her providers.

It explained why she had received limited benefit from treatment.

"Pain is not happening only to your shoulder," I said. "Pain is happening to you — to the entire being that is Michelle."

She was shocked. The idea that previous approaches to her pain and treatment had been so shortsighted was overwhelming to her. Along with her providers, Michelle had believed that she had only her physical injury to contend with.

Her shock was followed by a dawning revelation.

"Finally!" she said. "Finally I understand why my pain has seemed so mysterious!"

And then she began to cry again, this time tears of relief.

Michelle's journey with chronic pain is typical. My intake packet and initial meeting are intended to validate and articulate what most patients intuitively know — that chronic pain infuses and affects their entire being. This, often for the first time, grants them release from self-blame for not recovering, and from anger at their providers for failing them. It liberates them to release heroically held suffering, often, as with Michelle, in a powerful expression of sadness. They realize that they have always sensed the truth. That the information and treatments they have been receiving from their providers — despite those providers' years of dedicated research and practice — have missed the mark.

As I listen to a story like Michelle's and hear the litany of misunderstandings, the tales of untreated damage piled upon damage, *after* the initial physical injury, I feel grateful that I might offer hope. I am also angry that the condition has come to its current state. You might feel this way as well. It's painful to witness the consequences of failed or destructive surgeries, unsuccessful rehabilitation, and opioid dependence, knowing that these were potentially avoidable. So many pain problems need never have come to possess and control the person's entire life. And yet it happens. But take heart now — this is all correctable.

THE TREATMENT ENVIRONMENT

There are no villains in chronic pain treatment. The medical community works in expert, compassionate, and excellent ways to reduce suffering. I work collaboratively with many fine providers who appreciate and endorse the understanding offered here. Unfortunately, this approach has not yet been fully integrated into the treatment community at large.

Yet it is the way of human knowledge to evolve. At one time, healers used to believe mental illness was caused by evil spirits, and that making a hole in someone's head would release the spirits and cure them. Eventually, Sigmund Freud demonstrated that mental illness was neither demonic nor even purely biological but involves people's needs and desires.

In medicine, the discovery of unseen bacteria transformed the entire culture of health care. The history of healing is a testament to the commitment on the part of healers to seek deeper and different perspectives and understanding of suffering. In this light, providers and patients today may simply not know the true nature of what generates and perpetuates pain.

In my investigations of the mystery of chronic pain, I have learned from my patients and their providers — those who experience chronic pain themselves and those who bear witness to the experience — what that experience *means*. This individual experience holds the most crucial knowledge to help us learn how to manage and recover from chronic pain. The information is complicated and unique. It resides in the meaning of the pain in each person's life.

Redefining the Treatment Plan

During Michelle's first office visit, we discussed the findings from the extensive intake packet she had completed. It identified, among other things, loss or damage to many of her tasks, activities, and relationships. It identified challenges to her ambitions, goals, aspirations, and values. It revealed the creation of many new stressors in her life, which had undermined her ability to cope. These included major negative impacts to her self-esteem, work, career, relationships, physical conditioning, emotional state, and sense of identity.

> **"Ultimately, healing may require a personal transformation."**

Beyond just noting what had happened to Michelle's life, it was in discussing the personal meaning Michelle attributed to these negative events that revealed the extent to which she was affected by them. These impacts, taken all together and viewed holistically, rounded out the whole story. It was critically important that we view Michelle's pain from a sense of personal meaning.

With this perspective, we were able to partner in constructing a treatment plan to address each impact she had suffered, beginning with crisis intervention where needed, and moving on to permanent resolution. By following this new plan, Michelle was able to regain a sense of empowerment about managing her pain and treatment. And she gained the power to recapture lost aspects of her life. She also eventually learned how to evolve and maintain this approach and plan even without my help.

When my clients begin to understand the true extent and complexity of what has happened to them in their chronic pain, some feel overwhelmed. The authenticity of the information compels them to abandon the idea of a simple solution or cure. They recognize the challenge of what they'll need to know and what roles they will need to play to achieve successful outcomes.

Most importantly, my clients finally feel understood.

This helps them recognize that they need to become proactive in their own care at a level they had never contemplated. Most daunting, they realize that, ultimately, *healing may require a personal transformation.* This usually involves new and more effective ways of coping along with greater levels of emotional vulnerability.

My clients are not the only ones who feel overwhelmed. When their providers receive my reports, they realize that their every effort has been shortchanged by a profound lack of critical information about what their patient has been presenting to them. Providers too must abandon cherished notions about how pain should be understood and how care needs to be managed, given the realities of what they're up against.

Despite these challenges, both providers and patients are reassured because they finally have a roadmap to find their way out of the chronic pain wilderness. The analysis I provide reveals specific targets for treatment as well as techniques that show how the various damages can be eliminated or minimized Once you read this book and understand the concepts and techniques, you will be better able to assess your own challenges and guide your providers in helping you. You will be more able to develop the structure of your treatment needs. While you may not be able to practice full mastery just from a study of this book, you will be considerably more empowered with orientation and techniques to move toward thriving. Eventually, this can become a self-sustaining process.

I see the resulting reassurance demonstrated vividly in my clients' expressions of relief by the end of their first meeting with me. I hear it in the voices of their providers. Providers feel more empowered to plan their interventions based on a much deeper understanding of what their patients are experiencing and how that experience feeds back into the pain and response to treatment. They realize for the first time that critical information about their patients' pain will be disclosed and their suffering will be better understood.

These providers are now empowered to design care that serves their patients as individuals, and in an optimal way. They are grateful to be able to apply their expertise in a context that enables them to do their job more successfully. That context is a holistic understanding of who their patient is and what collateral damage is undermining diagnosis and recovery.

Centering Your Experience

Medical diagnosis and treatment are only the starting point of a holistic treatment approach. While medical treatment attempts to heal the damage from physical injury or disease, it doesn't necessarily treat the individual's sense of loss, difference, and diminution.

What I find people desire most profoundly is to live their lives to the fullest and to have their needs met. In the context of chronic pain, I must diagnose the person — the entire person — and their entire life. That is how I recognize what is essential to understand and treat in order to optimize medical treatment outcomes.

In my practice, this is accomplished by looking at what has happened to you since your injury, or since the onset of disease, and what is continuing to happen. I study your entire experience: How your injury has affected you both physically and personally. How the passage of time, your past, present, and future — in short, your life story — have affected the level of impact. Also, what you have experienced in the treatment environment. This approach leads to a truly individualized diagnosis and treatment plan.

THE TRUTH ABOUT CHRONIC PAIN

It is appalling to realize that neither the people experiencing chronic pain nor most of their providers — nor anybody else in their life — fully understand how they have been affected, let alone why they remain disabled and in pain. It's little wonder that I hear, repeatedly, "No one understands."

You're right: No one does.

But the truth of chronic pain *can* be assessed and understood. Further, the methods to ameliorate or even cure those impacts exist. The collateral damage done by pain and chronic disease creates threats to important needs. Unrecognized and untreated, this creates chronic suffering. When these damages and threats are recognized, however, they can be treated and either cured, marginalized, or minimized. Dispelling the mystery of chronic pain is the first step toward recovery.

> "Chronic pain is a system of harm created by the failure to treat all the damages created by unresolved pain."

In the next chapter, we'll look at where your own post-injury experience has caused damages to your life. It is essential to explore and attend to these damages, because these are what lead to the chronic crisis we call chronic pain. Chronic pain is a system of harm created by the failure to treat all the damages created by unresolved pain.

PERSONAL EMPOWERMENT

The process of personal empowerment begins with you and your providers engaging in an accurate and empathic exploration and understanding of your experience post-injury, across all dimensions of your life. This experience starts with the onset of your pain, followed by your entry into the medical system. It is crucial that you and your providers understand all the damage your pain has created in your life. Failing to do this creates the foundation, ironically, for disempowerment — for you as well as for your providers. But by dispelling the apparent mystery of your pain, you can bypass the highway to disability and move onto the road to empowerment and recovery.

Chapter 3

Injury and Collateral Damages

Chronic pain, as chapter 2 revealed, has many facets, and only one of them is physical. We have a medical system that is disproportionately focused on that one facet without sufficiently considering the collateral damages that can impact function, behavior, and meaning. Most of these collateral damages occur in three areas of your life:

(1) the physical, including physical harm caused by the injury and the post-injury pain — and "injury" can be to an internal system, such as the vascular or respiratory system, or can be caused by non-tangibles, such as postural habits that lead to restriction that lead to immobility and pain;

(2) the personal, or how your pain affects you as a person, as a unique individual with unique interpretations about what injury means to you in your life ; and

(3) the medical, meaning any harm you may experience in the course of seeing your doctors and receiving medical treatment. (Medical treatment may seem an unlikely source of additional damage, but it can happen, and there is even a specific term for it: *iatrogenic*, which can refer to something as simple as getting a rash from a prescribed cream or as drastic as having the wrong leg operated on.)

Parts 2, 3, and 4 go into much more detail on these three main areas, but this chapter offers an overview of how to approach, explore, and analyze your collateral damages. Undertaking this personal inquiry and assessment is the first step to recovery.

For many, this self-assessment includes facing hard truths about what has happened to you, but in such a way that you don't feel defeated.

Understand that acknowledgment of these hard truths is not resignation to them. Rather, acknowledging negative or discomfiting realities is the first step toward personal empowerment. And the pursuit of personal empowerment, including in how you cope and communicate, is the key to a return to your life, your independence, and a return to functioning. This short but important chapter is designed help you appreciate how complex chronic pain, given all the variables of an imperfect medical system, a complex body to begin with, and a unique self, and to begin to give you hope that there are ways to improve your situation in spite of these variables.

> "Acknowledging hard truths does not mean resigning to them. Rather, it's the first step toward personal empowerment."

THE TRIGGERING EVENT

In chapter 2, you learned to look at chronic pain as a natural disaster, like a hurricane. It is a triggering event with consequences.

If you break your arm, that is the initial event (the storm) that triggers other events (the collateral damages). A broken arm will trigger pain and discomfort, disruption to many of your regular activities, and possible emotional suffering and negative treatment experiences. These are just some of the effects on your life that naturally flow from being injured. When pain becomes chronic, this process continues to accumulate more and more significant impacts, with no apparent end. However, if you focus only on the initial physical damage, you are likely to perceive the initial event as the *only* problem, not as a *triggering event* that produces other ongoing challenges.

> "What happens when curative healing is hard to achieve, or not straightforward, or unobtainable?"

When you break your arm, it's set and put in a cast. Six weeks later, the cast is removed, you do physical rehabilitation exercises, and you're back to normal. If the damage to your body is identifiable, understood, and curable in a short amount of time, this may be enough.

Unfortunately, not all injuries and diseases are easily understandable, treatable, or curable. What happens when curative healing is hard to achieve, or not straightforward, or unobtainable? The resolution of your pain becomes less certain, and its power in your life becomes potentially more impactful. But does it need to be?

THE UNNECESSARY CONFUSIONS

When you think about how much pain you're in, why it hurts so much, why treatment doesn't seem to help, why you aren't getting better, do you feel confused? Do you encounter other people with the same injury who seem to suffer less than you do, or make more progress than you have? Situations like these become more understandable when you learn to identify collateral damages.

Stop and pay attention to how your pain affects what you can and cannot do.

Now, think about how you feel about these restrictions.

Does this help you recognize a bigger picture? Does it help you better understand why your pain feels the way it does, why it undermines your ability to function, why treatment does or doesn't help?

Injuries affect different bodies in different ways, and individual nervous systems vary quite a lot from person to person. People have different levels of pain tolerance and different

> "Pain damages your ability to function, and this is the core of your physical and emotional suffering."

levels of physical condition and health. Two people with similar injuries may in fact experience very different levels of pain and disability.

Suppose ten people have herniated discs. Their MRIs look about the same, but across those ten people, some may have zero pain and zero impact on functioning, while others experience ongoing agony and disability. The reason for these different experiences is that we are all unique. We are all different, often in significant ways, across physical, emotional, and psychological states at the time of an injury.

The central question is this: What is being triggered in you?

Your pain is the center of your problem, but not the only part that matters. Because pain damages your ability to function, and this is what is at the core of the downward spiral of physical and emotional suffering.

Damages to function include physical limitations and restrictions, excessive stress, important losses, emotional instability, and possibly even a challenge to your sense of who you are. Examples include not being able to work, exercise, interact with your children physically, be intimate with your partner, or socialize in the ways you enjoy. Any of these outcomes can cause emotional and psychological reactions that then create a feedback loop with your pain. That means your individual emotional and psychological reactions objectively increase your pain. This is why it's so important that treatment efforts be aimed not just at eliminating the pain but especially at dealing with what the pain triggers and undermines in your own unique, individual life.

THE ROLE OF PAIN PERCEPTION

The fact is, we are all different, and one individual may perceive the same situation, or be affected by the same situation, differently from another. This fact is often overlooked by those seeking to understand and treat chronic pain. But to understand and relieve your own physical suffering, it is essential to take this uniqueness — your uniqueness — into account. To truly understand your pain perception, your tolerance for it, how you as an individual perceive it.

> "To understand and relieve your physical suffering, it is essential to take your uniqueness into account."

For example, if I were at the scene of a horrible car accident, the sight of people's injuries might make me sick to my stomach. An experienced emergency medical technician probably wouldn't have the same reaction. Same situation, two very different perceptions.

To a certain extent, your pain perception is based on three things: how much pain you can tolerate, how important the injury is to your overall functioning, and how much the impacts of the pain affect what you care about. You might, perhaps, perceive a toothache as a minor event with little consequence in your life. Breaking an arm has greater potential to create collateral damage, and you will likely perceive and experience the event as more significant and impactful. But an event that paralyzes you will be experienced as potentially calamitous.

So, ask yourself: How does my injury affect me? How does it affect my life? How does it affect my needs? How have I responded to the losses and threats my injury creates?

Our needs are many, and often changing. But regardless of what needs we have, we want them satisfied. The more a need is related directly to functioning that supports survival, the more we crave satisfaction. If you believe your most important needs may not be satisfied, or cannot be satisfied, that belief will cause high levels of stress.

Collateral damage is about not just a specific impact, such as job loss, but also how that impact relates to your ability to provide for yourself — a basic need. Your interpretation of your pain includes your awareness of how it has damaged or may damage your ability to function. This combination is what you feel. And everything involved in this combination must be understood and properly treated.

How you experience pain is also affected by how you think about it. Suppose you say, "My pain is killing me!" or "The pain will never end!" or "I can't do any physical activities." Exaggerated or unconfirmed beliefs about your physical state are not necessarily true, and they increase the functional impact of your injury — and thus your emotional suffering. This additional stress adds to your sense of threat to your needs.

There's another important principle to consider in pain management: Pain doesn't always mean injury; hurt doesn't always mean harm. Several elements of chronic pain can produce pain that is not the direct result of your injury. Guarding and protecting behaviors, such as stiffening your body to prevent movement, moving hesitantly, or bracing yourself, often cause pain in parts of your body that you're using to reduce your initial pain. And unexplained pain, over an extended period, can rewire your neurological system so that you literally experience more pain or different pain even though your injury remains the same. This pain is caused not by the injury itself but by a faulty reaction in your nervous system.

> "Pain doesn't always mean injury; hurt doesn't always mean harm."

It is important to recognize this: There can be pain without injury; there can be pain that does not signal any potential to reinjure you. Pain is not a reliable guide to how much damage has been done, or how much to expect your functioning to be impaired.

Why do we need to be able to make these distinctions? When you're in pain, what you think and what you know to be the truth can either help lessen your concerns or make you more fearful and stressed. Accurate beliefs and understanding can help a great deal in recovery, while inaccurate assumptions will likely contribute to a downward spiral. This is why it's so important to gain accurate knowledge of what's happened to you, why it hurts, and how you — as an individual — experience it.

The holistic approach to treatment I outline in this book is more complex than traditional approaches. It requires a much greater degree of knowledge and understanding on your part, and greater collaboration and coordination in your care. However, with these aspects in hand, you will be more empowered to recover from your injury and the impacts of your pain.

THE COMPLEXITY OF YOU

As we've seen, then, chronic pain occurs within your existing physical structure and how you perceive it. It also relates to who you are, the current moment in your life, and what's going on in your life in general. This is determined by your current personal circumstances, history, personality, values, intelligence, skills, experience, education, and culture.

Pain occurs in the complexity of all you are, and within whatever meaning and value you attribute to what happens to you. This includes three personal elements. The first is your *experience*—what has happened to you because of your injury and chronic pain, and what you're concerned will happen next. This includes impacts on your daily life: your routines, chores, responsibilities, relationships, and activities; your psychological and emotional state; and your expectations.

The second element is your sense of *who you are*, in every aspect. For example, you may be a lawyer, dedicated to being hardworking and supporting your family. You may value honesty and integrity above all else. You may be an athlete and a creative person. Pain affects all aspects of who you are. Knowing this will help you understand and change how you experience pain and what makes it better or worse—for example, your values. If you are one who values ambition, achievement, or productivity, the ways your pain limits these will cause added stress if you don't find a way to honor them.

The third element is your *history*. Your injury and the events and experiences that follow write a chapter in the story of your life. It is important to also know how this affects your history, and possible succeeding chapters in it, for many reasons.

Your past matters. For example, providers often offer types of physical treatment that cause pain and tell people that it's for their own good. People who have experienced physical, sexual, or emotional abuse are likely to experience more distress in this situation. Any extra distress caused by your hidden history may increase your anxiety and anger during treatment. Or suppose you have difficulty trusting people or dealing with authority figures. Maybe you have a history of anxiety and depression or being vulnerable or highly self-sacrificial. Any strong reactions or strong emotions can limit the benefit you get from treatment such as physical therapy. They will have a negative effect on how you experience your treatment and how empowered you feel going through it. Truly, chronic pain cannot be understood without taking *you* into account.

Your personal history also encompasses how you satisfy your needs, how you determine your expectations and goals; it includes your emotional, spiritual, and psychological life and the strengths that help you deal with major challenges.

It's important to know all relevant aspects of your history and how they may be operating in your life. Your pain may be a major disruption in the continuity of your life's story thus far.

ALL THE NEEDS THAT NEED HEALING

An essential question for each person in pain is this: What needs to be healed for you? Answering this question begins with understanding how collateral damage affects your needs. Needs represent all that matters to you for survival; for your physical, emotional, psychological, and existential well-being; and for satisfying all your wants and desires, regardless of how essential they are. In many ways, needs are what make you who you are. Damage one need, and it can affect some — or all — of the others. For example, if pain causes you to lose your job, your need to provide for yourself is damaged. But that damage also may affect your self-esteem, or your marriage and your need to have a life partner.

Part of the reason chronic pain is so overwhelming is because it affects so many needs. When you face the possibility of losing what matters most to you, this may in turn undermine your emotional stability — your ability to cope and to be yourself. Harm or damage to your needs is a major contributor to your experience of pain. It becomes obvious, then, that this harm to your needs must be neutralized, resolved, or at least lessened. Your recovery must focus not just on your need to be physically healthy and pain-free but on addressing every other need that has been damaged and working to get them met more successfully. Chronic, incurable pain must be treated in ways that restore power to you, the whole person.

In other words, your whole life must be healed. The remaining chapters in this book will offer many strategies and techniques for addressing and satisfying your needs.

UNDERSTANDING THE SLOW TRAUMA

How many times have you felt that your pain was lessening, only to have another flare-up and feel like you're back to square one again? Once you've been injured, each new progression of the injury, or additional physical or life impact that follows, can complicate and compound the injury you began with, especially when it goes unrecognized and untreated. So it's essential to understand how ongoing and escalating life damage may be contributing to these setbacks. For example, a "typical" recovery from a herniated disc, based on statistics, is often undermined by the emotional crisis the pain and injury can create in a person's life, and then again by underestimating the stress of the too-slow recovery. This causes what I refer to as *slow trauma* — a series of events that accumulate to the level of trauma over time.

Let's return to the metaphor of chronic pain as natural disaster and consider what happened in Japan in 2011. It began with an earthquake. Over time, that earthquake was followed by a tsunami, flooded cities, damage to nuclear facilities, and thousands of deaths. These events caused profound displacements of populations and major economic impacts. Tainted water and food caused disease and long-term damage to people's health and welfare. We can clearly see that everyone caught in that disaster suffered multiple major losses, short-term and long-term.

The ultimate effect of this series of events included profound grief, huge adjustments, and a need to rebuild lives. But imagine that in this situation, the only impact anyone attended to was the original earthquake's damage to housing. If there had been no attention to the major crises in the other areas of damage, those crises, over time, could only have multiplied.

Chronic pain, like an earthquake, sends wave after wave of destruction into your life, resulting in major impacts to your needs. The more needs that are threatened or compromised, the more potential for that collateral damage to compound the original physical damage. This cycle exacerbates and perpetuates pain and inhibits your recovery.

We are wired to attend to and resolve all threats to any of our needs — it is a survival instinct. If we don't attend to these threats, or if we fail to resolve them, we enter a state of crisis — an unstable state of high tension and stress. Stress is a major contributor to pain, and the more stressed you are, the harder it is to cope. I hope you can now see that if the extensive impacts of pain on your many life needs remain unrecognized or untreated, they cause chronic stress. This is why stress management is often the focus of pain management counseling.

So, as you read about the physical impacts of chronic pain in part 2, please keep in mind what you've learned so far. In that section, physical impacts can be seen to be triggered not only by injury but also by the ongoing impact of pain on functioning; on your personal perception of events; on how they affect your life, your needs, and you as a person; and how they create emotional trauma over time. Untreated, these physical impacts can lead to ever-increasing stress and suffering.

Remember, acknowledging negative realities is the first step toward empowerment. There are many ways to minimize or eliminate the power of your particular collateral damages, which you will find in the various chapters of this book that are most relevant to you. Once these recovery strategies are revealed and understood, you can move toward healing — and thriving.

Tools and Takeaways for Part 2

Continuing with the work you may have started in part 1, you'll find the appendix A assessments will reveal hidden contributors to your pain and help you begin to identify what's most important to include in your recovery plan:

- Physical Impacts Inventory
- Post-Injury Physical Experience Inventory
- Emotional and Psychological Impacts Inventory
- Physical Impacts Checklist

Bottom Line

Chronic pain affects your physical state and physical needs, your physical functioning and physical identity. Acknowledging difficult realities is the first step toward empowerment. In addition, there are techniques that can prevent, mitigate, marginalize, or even undo many of the physical impacts of chronic pain.

PART 2

The Physical
Experience

Chapter 4

The Body Is the Setting

This chapter begins our exploration of how chronic pain creates physical damage beyond the initial injury. Because chronic pain is more than hurt and damage to your structure. It changes your body, your ability to function and get your needs met, and your emotional, psychological, and existential states.

These add to your pain and suffering. They also muddy the water, so to speak, and make it harder to understand the true levels of pain resulting from your injury. Most importantly, they limit the benefit you might receive from treatment. From sleep problems to limited mobility and activity, from loss of physical conditioning to loss of physical identity, the physical impact resulting from chronic pain affects your whole self.

For example, suppose your muscles are weakened and less flexible from lack of activity, or your immune system is weakened by the chronic stress that accompanies your pain. Or your concentration and attention are compromised, or your self-image is negatively changed. You may know these things are happening in a general sense, but you may not have paid significant attention to their impact. Without that attention, you won't know how they affect your pain and your success in treating that pain.

Becoming completely aware of your physical experience and physical impacts is the first step. In the chapters that follow, examine how each element interacts with your pain and undermines your functioning. This will help clear up any confusion you may have about how these are contributing to your pain. It will also maximize the benefit you get from medical treatments, especially if you and your providers are able to factor in and treat *all* of your current physical impacts. Your complete understanding will also give you a greater sense of the possibilities and opportunities you have to apply your own abilities and help yourself.

Let's say the physical damage from your original injury requires physical therapy. If your muscles have become weaker and less flexible due to lack of activity over time, you may also need physical reactivation and reconditioning to help you get full value from the physical therapy. This means your physical therapist will need to know your entire physical history, both before and since the injury occurred, including the specifics of your day-to-day physical changes and decline. They must take those changes in your physical state into account to determine how to make it more likely that their treatments and activities will help you, and how much.

I had a client once who, for almost three years after his back injury, spent 90 percent of his time lying down or in a recliner. This caused major physical atrophy, which in turn made it unlikely that a newly prescribed course of physical therapy would help him — unless he was physically reactivated and reconditioned first. Muscles that have become weak and atrophied require special treatment (read more about this in chapters 6 and 7). Unfortunately, neither my client nor his providers had paid much attention to this information, and so his physical therapy failed to help him.

When treatment fails, it's easy to develop fears of movement, pain, and re-injury, as well as to experience depression and perceived disability. It's easy to dwell on all the worst possible outcomes or catastrophize. If there is truly a limit to how much you can benefit from treatment, so be it. But if treatment fails merely from a lack of attention to collateral damages, I call that tragic.

Let's start by looking at the physical state your pain began in.

PHYSICAL RISK FACTORS

Chronic pain emerges within your body as it currently is. This is often complicated. Injuries often involve not just where you've been hurt but potentially all parts of your physical functioning. For example, if you already had a knee injury and now you have a back injury, that combination will complicate matters. A condition like high blood pressure, an auto-immune disorder, or diabetes will affect how you manage the stress caused by pain and how well your body can overcome the pain. Interactions like these are individual, variable, and often tricky to unravel.

Some aspects of physical makeup may interfere with recovery and make a person more susceptible to chronic pain. Factors like gender, age, health, weight, lifestyle, and diet are known to affect people's response to pain. Posture, sleeping patterns and position, and levels of stress and anxiety may increase or decrease the experience of pain. Lifestyle choices, like eating unhealthy foods or not exercising regularly, may add to the problem. And substance use, including smoking or alcohol dependency, also affects people's experience of and recovery from pain.

In other words, the condition of your overall health is relevant to your pain. You may have a weakened immune system that leads to frequent infections or illness. You may have existing or past health conditions that are difficult to treat, thus increasing stress, or that contribute directly to chronic pain. For example, conditions like endometriosis, ulcers, acid reflux, and urinary tract infections cause pain all on their own, separate from injury-related pain.

A person's hormonal balance can affect neuromuscular control and the strength and weight of muscles, tendons, and ligaments. Central nervous system adaptations affect how pain is processed. The endocrine system can also contribute: If someone's thyroid, hypothalamus, adrenal glands, or pituitary glands are overactive or underactive, this will affect how much pain they have. And there are many common health conditions that can affect pain by increasing inflammation in the body.

Given all the different variables in different people's bodies that can influence pain, functioning, and recovery, it becomes perhaps less surprising that efforts to diagnose and treat chronic pain sometimes get confused. I introduce these elements to help you understand the many things that affect chronic pain but are usually left out of addressing it. Understanding how any of these variables might affect you and contribute to your pain is an essential part of your story, and highly relevant to your approach to addressing your own chronic pain.

INJURY PLUS CONSEQUENCES

Like most people, I used to think that pain was simply a physical event. Almost immediately after I began my work in chronic pain management, though, I began to see the similarities between chronic pain and the chronic mental illness I used to work with on the hospital team. Just like with mental illness, pain seemed to be an event-plus-consequences to my patients. These added consequences are part of the setting pain and treatment occur in, just like risk factors. Over my years of practice, I began to catalog and then assess these consequences, and this is how I arrived at a crucially different understanding of what needs to be considered, accommodated, and treated, even on a purely physical level. Because understanding the consequences and successfully taking them into account can make the difference between someone's experience of unrelenting pain or reduced pain, as well as the difference between treatment failure, just surviving, or growing in life despite your pain.

I found it horrifying to discover all the unnecessary treatment failure and suffering that had occurred — and was still occurring. Most people I work with had not previously been aware of the different aspects of the consequences of their injury, starting at a physical level. How I wished people had been put on notice — from day one of their pain — to pay attention to this, to track and report it.

When I started my initial work in chronic pain management in a rehabilitation program, my first observations of the consequences of the injury were that pain affects people physically, beyond the initial pain and injury. This was, in part, because my background in the martial arts had made me more mindful of the physical consequences of an injury beyond the structural impact and pain. What followed was a growing awareness of how physical damage, pain, and loss can affect people cognitively, and in terms of stress. All of these added to the setting in which treatment occurs. Impacts in all of these areas will be addressed in the chapters that follow.

CHANGES IN EMOTIONAL AND PSYCHOLOGICAL STATES

Before you had chronic pain, your life probably had an order and a list of ingredients that defined you. These ingredients included a familiar and consistent physical, psychological, and emotional state. Now, because of the onset and continuation of pain, you've experienced significant changes to all of these states. It's important to pay attention to all of the changes and to learn how they can affect your pain and your recovery.

Part of the setting your injury occurs in is your psychological and emotional state at the time you were injured. You may have been very well balanced emotionally and psychologically. Your life may have been positive and well-ordered. Or you might be a person that has a number of different mental health issues or other situational issues and stressors in your life that made you less stable and vulnerable when the injury occurred. These are important variables to assess in understanding how your pain impacted you in the beginning. In addition, there are the changes produced in how you were at the beginning by the effect pain had on that state. Pain experiences change people's emotional and psychological states.

Let's look first at how your whole self can be undermined by your injury and persistent pain. In our metaphor of the natural disaster, we see that the disaster causes people, things, and much of what we value about ourselves to be lost. Someone who experiences chronic pain is like a person whose home has been inundated by a flood. The initial damage is physical but eventually challenges your emotional and psychological needs, and your life as you have known it is endangered.

Like most people in this situation, you're likely to focus your efforts on the physical damage — which in this case is the initial injury. You check to see if the house (your body) is livable and if anything can be salvaged. You try to save anything that you can, but you definitely suffer from the immediate losses: the pain resulting from the injury. Unfortunately, you can't always prevent further damage from unfolding — like treatment that fails to cure the injury, or coping skills that fail in the face of overwhelming stress. Over time, experiencing significant painful vulnerability can cause negative emotional and psychological consequences. In chronic pain, this level of collateral damage flowing from the physical impact of your injury is part of the *damage to your life*.

> "The longer the delay in finding a new normal, the greater the potential harm."

When collateral damages have accumulated to this extent, you are likely to suffer increasing losses and deprivations. Your ability to cope and to protect yourself from further harm — such as through professional treatment and personal coping mechanisms — may diminish as the conditions created by the "flood" fester and compound.

Eventually, you adopt a way of thinking where you try to acknowledge the harm that has been done and your limited ability to fix it. You may believe your suffering will go on and on and try to learn to accept it. This is the traditional treatment approach for chronic pain.

Indeed, your situation *will* get worse if time passes without attention to recovering or restoring your more stable and positive emotional and psychological states. Time passing in chronic pain can undermine this, like delays in rebuilding your home, restoring your finances, and attending to your physical and emotional health after a natural disaster. The longer the delay in finding a new normal, the greater the potential harm.

But now, by attending to all of the damage — not just the water damage from the flood but also the rot in the baseboards and the accumulating mortgage payments and the stress of not knowing what to do next — we've left the limited traditional approach to chronic pain behind. In the holistic approach presented in this book, your treatment plan will include all of the collateral damages and attention to improving as many areas as possible. We're looking at the harm you've experienced from the time of your injury and across time, for as long as it remains unresolved.

Many of the people I've worked with have been strong and persistent in their efforts to overcome their pain. But they didn't know it was import- ant to track and attend to the setting their pain occurs in, as described in this chapter, let alone all of the damages identified in the succeeding chapters, like sleep disruption and loss of physical strength and flexibility. After we worked together to document the extent of these, we worked all of these into an overall treatment plan that takes them into account, accommodates for them, and insures they don't interfere any more than is necessary, to allow for every area of their life to begin to improve. Truly, knowledge is power!

> "Attention to all the harm you've experienced is essential. Knowledge is power!"

So, how *do* you uncover all the harm done to your physical needs and functioning — by your original injury and by its collateral damages? In chronic pain, this is revealed through an analysis of your post-injury phys- ical experience and the dysfunction it includes. That's what the remaining chapters in part 2 address:

(1) Sleep disruption (chapter 5)
(2) Physical de-activation, including excessive downtime, avoidance behaviors, loss of ordinary movement, loss of task abilities, and guarding and protecting behaviors (chapter 6)
(3) Physical de-conditioning, including atrophy, energy loss, medical complications, damage to physical systems, weight loss or gain, and decreased pain tolerance (chapter 7)
(4) Cognitive impact (chapter 8)
(5) Chronic stress (chapter 9)
(6) Psychological implications, including the loss of physical identity (chapter 10)

Before you proceed with these chapters, you may want to use the self-assessment tools in appendix A to identify which of the many possible physical impacts apply to your experience. The self-assessment tools are intended to help you organize what's important to include in your recov- ery plan. Keep in mind that for each impact identified and described in each chapter, the Recovery sections show you how to prevent, minimize, or better manage them.

The goal is not to make it seem as if you have even more problems than you already knew, but rather to give you the opportunity to empower yourself in your recovery by eliminating these impacts as contributors to your pain. You do this by identifying, naming, and embarking on recovery strategies that help you move toward healing — and thriving.

COGNITIVE IMPACT

Part of the setting pain occurs in is your current memory, attention, concentration, self-control, mental flexibility, and responsiveness — a set of skills and capacities often called *executive function*. These cognitive impacts affect your ability to function in an optimal way at a "hardware" level, psychologically and emotionally. This is especially true if your neurological system gets rewired (for example, with complex regional pain syndrome; for more about this, see chapter 13, "Functional Impacts").

Cognitive impairments make it hard to process and accommodate the multiple negative impacts caused by your pain. They compound emotional suffering and stress and increase your pain. It's hard enough to acknowledge the reality of losses you've suffered, let alone overcome them, when you cannot attend to them, think about them, or effectively address the problems. You'll learn more about cognitive and stress related impacts in chapter 8, "Cognitive Impacts," and chapter 9, "Chronic Stress."

Throughout the remaining six chapters in part 2, I will identify and describe multiple possible physical impacts of chronic pain in detail. More importantly, the Recovery sections at the end of each chapter will offer many possible ways to neutralize or eliminate — or, at the least, more effectively master — these impacts.

Chapter 5

Sleep Disruption

S leep-disrupted nights might as well be considered normal for people living with chronic pain: 50 to 90 percent of people with chronic pain report not sleeping well. Sleep disruption includes both loss of quality and loss of hours of sleep. These can result from difficulty falling asleep, frequent awakening during the night and trouble getting back to sleep, awakening earlier than desired, and non-restorative sleep. Insomnia is the most frequent sleep problem associated with pain. Chronic pain is a distraction that is hard to turn off.

Solving this problem often requires overcoming long-held habits, which can be physically and emotionally difficult as well as create new and different physical problems. For example, one of my clients with back pain had to learn to sleep propped on a pillow, in a half-sitting position, after a lifetime of sleeping on his side. This was so difficult for him that he turned to sleeping medications and began to overuse his opioids, which further undermined his quality of sleep and his daily functioning.

The significance of sleep disruption to chronic pain is well documented. Sleep disruption can, all by itself, increase your pain — by up to 50 percent. It can also cause other collateral damage, as described later in this chapter. But I've found that not everyone has been fully informed about the impact of sleep disruption, let alone been comprehensively treated for it. This chapter names the major impacts of sleep disruption: to pain sensitivity, daily functioning, and mental acuity. The Recovery section offers multiple approaches to minimize, eliminate, or better manage these impacts.

EFFECT ON SLEEP QUALITY

Pain does not just make it hard to get to sleep, it makes your sleep lighter and more easily subject to awakening. If pain wakes you up, you might lose the restorative state of sleep in which you dream. This, in turn, may increase your sensitivity to pain. Further, we all have a body clock. The tissues and organs in your body operate according to biological rhythms. The body clock keeps this process running according to schedule. It regulates the processes of sleeping, eating, and temperature. Meanwhile, many pain medications are known to interrupt or affect sleep. Codeine, morphine, and other opioids can cause insomnia. Opioid pain medications can also cause sleep apnea. Sleep disruption can also arise with antidepressants, muscle relaxants, nerve-related medications, and anti-inflammatory medications.

When you do not feel rested and refreshed by a night's sleep, you may experience diminished energy, a depressed mood, fatigue, and increased pain during the day.

EFFECT ON PAIN SENSITIVITY

Loss of sleep of any kind makes you more sensitive to pain — it lowers your pain threshold and pain tolerance, making your existing pain feel worse. It does this by causing increased production of inflammatory chemicals in the body called *cytokines*. Sleep disruption can also cause more anxiety, anger, and depression, and these emotions, in turn, can also increase pain.

EFFECT ON DAILY FUNCTIONING

It's important to remember that when sleep is disrupted by chronic pain, pain is not the only problem. It also undermines your ability to function. And undermined functioning leads to other collateral damage.

Sleep disruption directly causes a loss of energy, which makes it tougher to be active and exercise. Among other things, this often leads to weight gain, which can further restrict exercise. In addition, weight gain can lead to sleep apnea, which prevents a restful night's sleep.

Other impacts from sleep disruption include increased proneness to accidents, slowed response time, inattention, impaired judgment, disorganized thinking, poor fine and gross motor control, slurred speech, clumsiness, difficulty bringing eyes into focus, difficulty recognizing objects by touch, and difficulty vocalizing an idea or piecing together a sentence. Sleep disruption also damages both short-term and long-term memory.

When you cannot escape your pain through sleep, you cannot rest, reenergize, or relax. This is likely to make you feel more trapped in your pain, more damaged, more tortured by it. Lack of sleep can even produce mental illness, such as perceptual problems and paranoia, depression, and anxiety disorders.

EFFECT ON MENTAL ACUITY

While you sleep, your brain normally orders, integrates, and makes sense of things that have happened to you. It locks in memories, new learnings, and new skills. When there is sleep disruption, this brain work may not occur. Attention skills are affected too. If you haven't gotten enough sleep, you cannot pay attention to anything as well as you normally would. Someone in an intensely sleep-deprived state may not be able to remember a few digits of a telephone number, let alone perform any complex tasks. If you notice yourself going around in circles while attempting to complete tasks, it may well be that you have some level of sleep deprivation.

> "Chronic pain demands that you innovate and create new strategies, skills, and habits that aid your recovery."

Brains that are sleep-deprived are less efficient. The ability to plan or coordinate actions can be temporarily impaired. If you haven't been sleeping well, you may notice you've lost the vital ability to effectively decide when and how to start or stop tasks. This can be a major challenge, especially if your daily functioning is already impaired by pain.

Because sleep-deprived brains easily get stuck in loops of activity or fogs of indecision, sleep-deprived people often find it hard to make plans or control how and when they take action. Instead, they fall back on the brain's automated systems. In other words, habit takes over, and you come to rely more heavily on repeating the same actions in the same situations.

This is bad news when it comes to bad habits. For example, people who are sleep-deprived eat more junk food. This is also bad news with respect to the creativity and innovation you need to assess and overcome your limitations. Sleepy people often feel incapable of changing their game plan. They are more likely to take ill-advised risks and less able to benefit from experience. In short, the effects of lack of sleep may get you stuck in strategic ruts.

It is vitally important to understand that chronic pain demands you be creative and adaptive. To manage it well, you need to create new strategies, skills, and habits that aid your recovery.

RECOVERY: SLEEP RESTORATION

It can be scary and overwhelming to think of how much collateral damage can be created by just one physical impact: sleep disruption. But the first step to recovery is simply to recognize how much you might be affected by any trouble you have sleeping at night. Fortunately, there are also numerous treatment options, for many types of sleep disruption, that can reduce or even eliminate the problem. Here are four strategies to start with.

Protect Your Sleep

As we just discussed, you cannot afford to have disrupted sleep if it can be at all avoided. Although medications to help you sleep are a common approach, they often cause more problems than they solve. Any use of painkillers or sleeping pills should be supervised by a physician and should take into consideration how they might actually add to the problem. Meanwhile, there are many common-sense and practical approaches to preventing sleep disruption, as well as more sophisticated approaches.

A simple first step, both straightforward and helpful, is to learn about and practice good sleep hygiene. Good sleep hygiene includes these essential practices:

- Make sleep a higher priority than other activities.
- Try to avoid emotionally upsetting conversations and activities right before you go to sleep.
- Establish a regular, relaxing bedtime routine or ritual. For example, take a warm bath, eat a light snack, or read for a short time just before bedtime.
- Watch your sleep timing: Try to go to bed at night and get up in the morning at the same time every day.
- Associate your bed with sleep: Do not get into bed until you are ready to fall asleep.
- Use the best pillows and mattresses you can find.
- Avoid stimulants such as caffeine, nicotine, and alcohol too close to bedtime. Also avoid eating large meals close to bedtime.

Additionally, the following strategies and daily habits can provide additional sleep hygiene support:

- Monitor your medications to see if they could be part of the problem.
- Consider taking melatonin. Melatonin is a naturally occurring brain hormone that works differently than sleeping pills.

- Research dietary practices that might either help or harm your sleep problems. WebMD is a good resource for this information. In general, a diet that supports sleep is similar to one that supports overall health: It includes nutrition-dense foods and limits foods that are higher in added sugars, saturated fat, and sodium.
- Avoid napping during the day.
- Ensure adequate exposure to natural light during the day — light exposure helps you maintain a healthy sleep-wake cycle. Also, consider light therapy, which helps treat a mismatch between your internal clock and your environment.
- Avoid drinking a lot of any type of liquid before bedtime, to minimize trips to the bathroom.
- Use your sleep time well. Try to use your time in bed constructively even if you can't fall or stay asleep. If you wake during the night, do not toss and turn and ruminate on things that worry or bother you. Instead, take this opportunity to meditate, listen to music or other soothing sounds with headphones, or find other more pleasant things to think about.

Use Bedtime Relaxation Techniques

Quieting down your environment for sleep, as recommended for good sleep hygiene, can, ironically, cause problems if pain is the only experience left to capture your attention. People experiencing chronic pain often report that one of their primary pain management tools during the day is distracting themselves by staying busy with other tasks, such as reading, watching television, engaging in hobbies or crafts, working, or conversing and interacting with others. But when you're trying to fall asleep, there are ordinarily no other distractions available to focus on. Because of this, you may perceive your pain as actually increasing right at the time you're trying to fall asleep. The longer it takes to fall asleep, the more stressful this situation becomes. However, there are solutions.

When you're in bed and it seems that pain is the only thing left to pay attention to, try practicing relaxation techniques, which can include meditation, breathing techniques, and creative visualization. Many people have told me they find meditation difficult and challenging and think they need help with proper technique. I point out that lying in bed wide awake is a perfect opportunity to practice. It's like free time.

I usually have my clients start with an easy form of meditation: progressive visualization. For this, you imagine a scene you associate with relaxation, such as a sunny beach or a mountaintop. Your task is to experience the scene with all your senses: seeing it, hearing the sounds associated with it, taking in the smells, the physical sensations. Try for virtual reality! Steady abdominal breathing is your meditation anchor and is helpful in this practice as well as with other meditation techniques. Use your breathing pattern to calm and focus your mind, then proceed with your meditation practice. Come back to the breathing if you're having trouble with the meditation.

The practice of meditation can reduce pain and stress, which helps promote restorative sleep. It can also affect the pattern of your sleep, resulting in more restful sleep, and help to quiet pain and anxiety when you're awake at night. Meditation may develop parts of the brain that help regulate physical health and pain perception.

Apply Anti-Anxiety Knowledge

Anxiety often contributes to difficulties falling asleep and can certainly make it hard to go back to sleep after you awaken during the night. One strategy to counteract anxiety is to journal each day during the early evening.

In your journal, write down every situation, personal and work-related, that's making you anxious. Score each on a 0 to 10 scale, with 10 being the highest level of anxiety. (A 10 is usually a life-endangering moment, like if you're about to be hit by a bus.) Be sure to check how important the issue is for you as an individual before rating it on the scale. For example, a life-threatening situation, a threat to a relationship, a threat to the welfare of a loved one, or a threat to your self-esteem are likely more important than being stuck in traffic.

Next, deliberately work to reduce your anxiety on each item, using all your coping and problem-solving skills. These will be discussed in more detail in chapter 15, "Operating-System Impacts." The more you can reduce your anxiety on all or most items, the less chance they will plague you when you're falling asleep or when you awake in the night.

Develop Supportive Physical Habits

Some common-sense and practical approaches to lessening pain or discomfort can also reduce sleep disruption. For example, use a heating pad (for muscular pain) or ice pack (for inflammation) at bedtime. Learn best practices for use of pillows and sleep supports and adopt proper positions for sleeping. The following activities can also be helpful:

- Vigorous exercise done four to eight hours before bedtime has been shown to help improve sleep quality. It may also help reduce anxiety, which can be a factor in sleeplessness.
- Yoga uses stretches and breathing exercises that promote psychological relaxation and reduced muscle tension, both of which aid better sleep.
- Acupuncture treatments stimulate nerves throughout the body to reduce pain and can also stimulate your level of nighttime melatonin.
- Biofeedback sessions use devices that can help you learn to control body functions like heart rate, muscle tension, and temperature, all of which can help you sleep.

Chapter 6

Physical De-Activation

P hysical pain and traditional pain treatment typically join together to launch a cycle of general physical deactivation — avoidance of movement and habits of excessive downtime, among others listed below. These behaviors may be understandable and even necessary, but there is a price to be paid for them, especially if you ignore their consequences. As part of acknowledging negative realities in chronic pain, it is critically important that you become completely aware of your physical experience and the full scope of your physical impacts in order to learn how to heal and thrive. Let's look at the detail, scope, and subtleties of physical deactivation, which are often missed or misunderstood.

LOSS OF ORDINARY MOVEMENT

Chronic pain, by definition, makes it hard to move comfortably. It can change the way you engage in your most ordinary and important everyday physical movements. You may start avoiding specific movements or becoming excessively cautious and physically tense. It's a common experience in chronic pain to misperceive the degree of your physical limitations and risk, and if you do, you'll likely choose, consciously or unconsciously, to become guarded or progressively less active, with the goal of avoiding any and all pain and additional harm.

Overall, it's important to distinguish *hurt* from *harm*. Pain doesn't always equate to damage or harm — for those who have suffered chronic pain, this is often hard to understand. However, if you assume that all pain, or hurt, means harm, it may cause you to shrink away even from beneficial treatment if it comes with some level of pain.

But I can attest that people's self-imposed restrictions on movement can be significant. They can range from minor hindrances to major impacts on your daily life. They can affect your ability to do things others take for granted, like lifting groceries, walking, climbing stairs, standing, bending, reaching, holding things, and even doing personal hygiene activities such as showering and washing your hair. Such restricted movement may hinder your ability to enjoy your life or be the person you want to be. It can also increase physical de-conditioning (discussed in chapter 7, "Physical De-Conditioning"), atrophy, and stress, which will further diminish activity, undermine treatment goals, and increase pain.

> "Under good guidance, you may discover that you are much safer than you imagine."

That said, movement should be approached with reasonable caution. People with chronic pain often injure themselves by attempting certain physical activities prematurely. And each new injury can reduce your activity level even further. Indeed, whenever possible, it is critical to obtain accurate medical information and professional guidance on how to calibrate your physical efforts. The best programs teach people to move in ways that are ergonomically correct and sustainable for them. Under good guidance you may discover that you are much safer than you imagine, more capable of movement and activity than you might have anticipated.

LOSS OF TASK ABILITIES AND RESPONSIBILITIES

It's also common for people with chronic pain to modify or abandon many of their usual tasks because of the pain. Tasks, habits, and routines that most people take for granted may become like Olympic events for you. You may have had to lower your standards for getting things done—and for doing them well. There are many reasons for this. You may be afraid to fail at a task. You may not want to be reminded of your new limits or risk pain or negative emotional flare-ups. All of this will push you to avoid making effort, and this in turn further weakens the body.

Task loss can include loss of the ability to carry out household chores, work responsibilities, and things you do in other roles in your life. Task loss also contributes to negative psychological impacts. What used to be so ordinary and easy for you has—at least temporarily—become out of reach. You may find your self-worth plummeting when you watch others doing chores or work tasks that you can't do anymore. You may feel envy. You may feel guilty about others doing things for you and fear that they will feel overburdened and reject you in turn. As time goes by, you may find that your inability to do your usual tasks does indeed cause inter-personal friction and resentment from those picking up the slack. (These psychological and emotional impacts will be more thoroughly covered in chapter 10, "Psychological Challenges.")

At the same time, task responsibilities you have let go of may be replaced by newly necessary tasks, often negative and stressful, like dealing with insurance companies and government agencies and the bureaucracy of the medical system. In fact, the ramifications of task loss can snowball rapidly. The Recovery sections in this and the next chapter include infor-mation and strategies to help you regain your tasks. But first we'll finish discussing the various aspects of physical de-activation.

USE OF AVOIDANCE AND DOWNTIME BEHAVIORS

People who have chronic pain often try to lessen their pain by sitting or lying down more often than usual. You probably do this too — and it makes sense! It's likely a conscious effort to avoid activities that can make your pain flare up. It's also behavior that's likely been reinforced by your provider's warning to "stop when it hurts."

While we all do whatever we can to get relief from pain and suffering, it's important to understand how inactivity can cause unwanted side effects and affect functioning. When you sit or lie down for extended periods of time, or avoid physical activity, your muscles change. For example, when the big muscles meant for movement — like those in your legs — are frequently immobile, this causes physical problems. Your hip flexors and hamstrings may shorten and tighten; the muscles that support your spine may become weak and stiff. These effects will make it increasingly difficult for you to engage in physical activity and thus to feel productive, needed, and useful. Downtime also has significant negative emotional impacts. How do you think your self-esteem will be affected, even though your pain is dictating your inaction, if you see yourself as the ultimate couch potato?

In summary, downtime may reduce your pain in the short term, but you will pay for it, over time, in loss of your ability to function, which most people say is the most stressful part of living with chronic pain. Learning how to move safely and tolerate reasonable discomfort will serve you well.

USE OF GUARDING AND PROTECTING BEHAVIORS

It's an understandable reality that you will adjust your body in whatever ways reduce or eliminate your pain. Protection from pain is a primary need, and living with chronic pain and the associated physical limitations can make the simplest of movements painful and traumatic. To avoid this, you may change the way you walk or sit, the way you hold and carry yourself, and the way you move. This is called *guarding and protecting*. Yet while adjustments and adaptations may need to be made, there's a price to pay. Because the physical accommodations you're making aren't always *conscious*, even those that often violate proper body mechanics.

Having worked with several thousand clients, as well as working with providers and reviewing their medical notes, I can say that people are often shocked when they first become aware of the scope and extent of the physical adjustments they've been making. Ironically, instead of reducing pain, these adjustments often exacerbate it and have the potential to create new problems as well.

Guarding behaviors may include stiffness, limping, bracing a body part, holding part of the body in an unnatural position, shifting weight away from the pain, over-relying on one side of the body, and flinching. Do any of these sound familiar to you? Guarding behaviors may also include facial expressions and verbalizations, such as cries, grunts, moans, grimaces, or huffs and puffs.

Protecting behaviors are meant to physically protect you against pain and may include avoiding contact with a particular body area, protecting the injured area by favoring it, intentionally limiting use or movement, and using a prosthetic, such as a cane, sling, brace, or walker. These behaviors are aimed not just at avoiding pain but also at reducing the fear of increasing the pain, causing re-injury, or experiencing negative emotional impacts. When these behaviors occur regularly over the course of time, they can easily add negative physical impact and loss of functioning, as well as exacerbate the original injury.

Let's look at an example. Neil was a client of mine who'd had minor foot surgery that resulted in chronic pain, largely due to Neil's own actions. Usually, wearing a foot boot is prescribed for the first six weeks after surgery. Without his doctor realizing it, Neil wore his boot for almost a year. Beyond that year, he also used crutches and a cane, without direction, advice, or counsel from his providers, for almost another whole year.

These behaviors created major atrophy in Neil's foot, ankle, and leg, which, in turn, created chronic pain and dysfunction where there hadn't been any before, entirely separate from the original pain leading up to the surgery or the immediate post-surgery pain. Neil's guarding and protecting behaviors also created pain in his neck that was directly related to the compensatory pattern he'd developed by working around his foot. His providers didn't understand what had created or was maintaining the neck pain, so his neck became a second chronic pain problem.

Once Neil and his providers understood his history of guarding and protecting behaviors and how they had created additional physical problems, he was able to work to remedy those problems and achieved a significant level of recovery.

Then there's Laura's story. After multiple back surgeries, she'd been out of treatment for several years, but she went back to physical therapy on the advice of her new doctor, who hadn't assessed her recent activity pattern. On the first physical therapy visit, Laura had a major pain flare-up, which caused everyone — herself, her therapist, and her doctor — to determine her case inappropriate for physical therapy. On investigation, however, I discovered that Laura had spent the previous two years lying on her side on a couch for 80 to 90 percent of every day. This had contributed to a major level of physical de-conditioning and atrophy, which was the actual reason for her reaction to physical therapy. Once I explained this to Laura and her providers, she was prescribed a physical re-activation program. Several months later, she was able to attend all her physical therapy sessions without flare-ups. This resulted in a significant reduction in pain and overall improvement in her functioning.

And here's an example of guarding behaviors that may not be obvious to you or your providers.

Abby, age twenty-nine, had suffered rib and neck cervical injuries when run over by a truck. Her injuries required fusion surgery on her back. The surgery was successful, and her cervical pain post-surgery was tolerable and expected.

Before the accident, Abby had been an athlete who played softball at a near-professional level. Eighteen months after surgery, she began to experience severe pain in her rib area when twisting her torso while playing softball or golfing. None of her providers were able to discern any physical cause for this pain, which had become quite disabling. She was referred to me by providers who suspected it was "psychological."

An extensive activity analysis of Abby's post-accident behaviors and activities revealed the truth. Though none of her providers were aware of it, Abby had avoided turning her torso or exercising her upper body for the eighteen months post-surgery — "to be safe." At the end of those eighteen months, she returned to playing softball, but without any re-conditioning of her upper body or gradual reintroduction of torso-turning movements.

Once she began to have the new pain, she went into physical therapy, where her therapist also failed to consider Abby's guarding and activity history. As Abby's pain worsened, she became fearful of turning her torso, and for the next year she avoided it like the plague, discontinuing most exercise. Once her providers became aware of her almost *three years* of guarding behavior, her physical therapist worked to first undo the physical atrophy this behavior had created. Within six months, Abby was able to turn and twist without significant pain.

So now let's talk about what you can do to recover from the physical de-activation related to your chronic pain.

RECOVERY: PHYSICAL RE-ACTIVATION

Personal transformation is the path from surviving to thriving. Physical impacts do not just cause more pain, they diminish you. Understanding this can motivate you to avert and defeat the damages of deactivation.

> "It begins with understanding that you are not powerless, and you are not helpless."

This will require many changes in how you operate — again, physically, emotionally, *and* psychologically. And all these changes are absolutely in your best interest.

The ideal scenario is to prevent physical collateral damages such as loss of ordinary movement and tasks, excessive downtime and activity avoidance, and guarding and protecting behaviors. Some of this is possible if you are aware of the issues and of all the preventive interventions you can use. If you cannot prevent the behavior or damage, however, there are also many techniques that can mitigate, marginalize, or even undo many aspects of physical deactivation. The section you are about to read provides techniques useful for both prevention and mitigation!

This approach begins with understanding that you are not powerless, and you are not helpless. You get to choose how you respond to the challenges you are faced with. The many techniques and approaches outlined below will be of greatest value once you have become aware of the cost of both the pain impacts, as outlined above, and the counters for them, outlined here. While much of this section on recovery from physical deactivation is derived from common sense, client reports, and clinical practice, some strategies require a deeper understanding of who you are and how you operate to get your needs met. Following are twelve strategies for recovery.

Assess Your Risk of Reinjury

All of my clients agree that if they had to make a choice, they would choose to forsake pain reduction if certain approaches would instead allow them to remain functional, active, and physically fit. Put yourself in a position where you can make that choice by assessing your risk comprehensively. This includes using your own research to complement that from your providers. (I will discuss this type of research in more detail in part 4.)

Essentially, you need to assess the distinction between pain and injury. This may require an extensive investigation. However, once you have this understanding, you will be much less likely to unnecessarily deactivate (through excessive downtime, avoidance of activities and ordinary movement, and guarding and protecting behaviors).

So before you begin to apply any of the recommendations in this section, it's essential to get adequate information — comprehensive information — from your providers. Find out exactly what your actual structural limits and risks are. Get specific directions on what is safe for you to do and what is not:

- Ask for careful clarification when providers tell you to stop your activities.
- Follow the treatment plan you and your provider agree upon only after you feel fully informed and are in common understanding.
- Ask questions about prognosis from all your providers. Get their benchmarks for your progress in recovery.
- Find out as much as you can about your type of chronic pain and its treatment to be sure that the limit to your functioning is not self-imposed.

In addition to a thorough questioning of your provider, there are a few simple ways to begin to understand the meaning of your pain as you experience it. Some information may be built into the pain itself. For example, the words you use to describe your pain may offer clues about what structure is generating it. Muscles, bones, and nerves each have their own unique descriptors, which have potential diagnostic value. *Sharp* suggests muscle pain. *Achy*, *sore*, or *dull* pain points to structural inflammation. Pain described as *burning*, *shooting*, or *electric shock* could be nerve-related.

Treatment interventions may also target specific structural areas. What portion of your pain do they affect? What percentage is muscle-, inflammation-, or nerve-related? Be sure to track this information and consider the value of this data. Pain management is most effective when it is based on reliable, verifiable data. Not all data needs to be highly technical — some is just based on common sense and your own good intelligence.

However, I cannot emphasize enough how important it is for you to have objective data to use as a basis for feeling safe and being secure in your physical actions. Whenever possible, it is critical to obtain accurate medical information and professional guidance on how to calibrate your physical efforts. A lack of this knowledge is at the center of many recovery failures. Once you are secure in the knowledge that the movements you undertake won't harm you, it becomes much easier to apply other approaches to counter physical de-activation.

Practice Body Awareness

Practice body awareness to minimize guarding behaviors. Guarding and protecting behaviors become deeply ingrained habits the body adopts over time in reaction to pain.

To counter physical guarding and protecting with awareness, periodically check the level of physical tension caused by your pain. Be mindful of how your body is reacting to your pain. For example, do you put more weight on your left leg because your right knee hurts? Do you clench your jaw? Hold your breath? Notice the extent of what you're doing physically to offset the pain. Ask yourself: Can I avoid compensating this way? Evaluate the things you are doing to escape your pain and discomfort. Ask yourself if they are an absolute necessity. Are there alternatives that have less negative impact?

This technique requires that you be knowledgeable about the structural mechanisms that generate your pain and about how your choice of physical behaviors affects you. For instance, you may be adding to the physical atrophy in the leg you are favoring. You may be creating a problem in your good leg. Protecting behaviors can reduce strength and mobility and undermine functioning.

The clients and providers I've worked with over the years have taught me ways that conscious effort can be made to reverse protecting behaviors. Beyond increasing body awareness, you can learn to re-teach your body how to carry out more appropriate patterns of physical behavior — patterns that relieve pain without unwanted side effects. Physical therapists and trainers can show you how to use strengthening and stretching exercises and educate you concerning proper body mechanics to help you correct how you have modified your movements to relieve pain.

You might become anxious when you work at changing these patterns that you believe have been protecting you from pain. If so, stress reduction techniques can help. Becoming more knowledgeable about the structural mechanisms that generate your pain will help reduce your anxiety too. The body operates as a balanced system, and physical therapy and occupational therapy professionals can help bring your body function into better balance.

Adjust to the New Normal

People with chronic pain have a tendency to avoid evidence of their limitations. But acknowledging your limitations is necessary to begin to deal with them constructively. You might see the need for this when you can't easily do the laundry without pain, or mow the lawn, or cook — so you avoid even trying. Unfortunately, many people think that modifying the way they do tasks is "giving in to the pain."

> "Don't fall victim to constantly comparing yourself to your past self. Work with what you've got."

Here is the truth: *not* doing what you want to, in any shape or form, is conceding that your pain has control of your life. If you do that, you add to your sense of helplessness.

Recovery from chronic pain means finding a way to thrive, no matter what the challenge is that you face. Having chronic pain does not mean that you cannot live life in any normal sense. Think of your current physical circumstances as your "new normal," and adjust accordingly. Instead of constantly comparing yourself to your past physical self, work with what you've got. There is no reason the "new normal" you seek has to be less than your previous life. (See chapters 11–14 for more about creating a "total" new normal, one that includes day-to-day functioning situationally and existentially and that reveals, respects, and accommodates the psychological and emotional damage your need for a new normal creates). Begin each day with the intention to live your physical life as fully as possible. Decide how you want to perceive and react to the changes that pain has caused in your physical and emotional life. How do you think about it? For example, is your pain dangerous and limiting by definition? Has it reduced your physical life, or is it challenging you to live?

You have an understandable need to seek pain relief. Is there an alternative to de-activation? Yes. The answer is to seek out choices, alternatives, that minimize de-activation and may even enhance your physical activities.

Proceed Like an Athlete

A great concept for achieving an enhanced new normal is to treat life as an athletic event. Take time to stretch and warm up before any important chore or activity, especially those known to cause flare-ups (such as extended sitting or standing, mowing the lawn, doing the laundry, preparing a meal, house cleaning, or washing the car). Do a formal cooldown after the activity.

It may seem contradictory, but in thinking like an athlete and looking at life as an athletic event, you may be able to minimize your physical de-activation and maintain or even improve your overall physical condition, despite your pain. Try to consider all physical activities as training sessions or athletic events. Prepare, approach, assess, recover. Activate, rather than de-activate, within your own known limits.

> "In every typical chore, there is an opportunity to strengthen the parts of the body involved."

This strategy includes any stretch or movement that can help your body transition from working hard to hardly working, without ill effects. Think about the way you engage in ordinary movement and use it to serve your activation goals. In every typical chore, there is an opportunity to strengthen the parts of the body involved. When turning a doorknob, for example, or opening a door, use that muscle tension to improve the strength in your wrist and forearm. Walk up the stairs in a manner that strengthens your legs, using good form and intention. Intentionally engage your abdominal and lower back muscles before getting up from or sitting down into a chair. Change your attitude toward activity from avoidance to finding opportunity. This will positively affect your physical condition and energy levels. In fact, this approach can preserve and even increase functioning, which in turn provides positive emotional energy.

Remember, all physical activities are potentially exercise.

Create an Adjustable Plan

Another way to counter de-activation is to establish a cascade of fallback alternatives for accomplishing something. I call this Plan A-B-C-D-E. Rather than setting yourself up for failure with a Plan A that may exceed your abilities on some days, make an adjustable plan, in advance, to help ensure that you will do something each day that contributes to your physical re-activation.

For instance, if your Plan A on a given day is to walk a mile, but it's not always possible, your Plan B might be to walk half a mile. If that's not possible, your Plan C might involve walking indoors on a treadmill, and so on. This way, if you find yourself unable to carry out what you had hoped to do, you don't have to abandon your plan: You can take on some less demanding version of it and still claim a success. You may not be able to cook on a particular day, but perhaps you can manage to do the laundry. Even lying down to rest, with intention, may be on your list of things you

> "Rather than reducing movement, activities, or tasks, plan them to be doable."

can do. Wherever possible, find a way to keep up some level of activity that supports recovery.

Note that adjustable plans work best when you are willing to make adjustments in both quality and quantity. Take every activity as a chance to be creative and efficient in getting things done. You might have to change the way you conceptualize chores. Modify or redesign how tasks get accomplished. Try to do things in a way where you're likely to increase your activity — even slightly. For example, if standing is too painful, cook sitting down, using a chair with wheels. Do your laundry in smaller loads. Use your best problem-solving skills and be creative in maintaining your functioning. For example, create a laundry chute to avoid having to lift too much. When you find the most efficient way of doing a task, it will become less taxing physically and leave more energy for other tasks.

In other words, rather than seeing yourself as falling short of your goals, activities, or tasks, plan them to be doable, even though differently done. If mowing the lawn is a physical impossibility, think about how you might do it in pieces on a rotating schedule. Or if your aim is to just be active each day, find a task with equal value that you don't ordinarily do, like cooking a meal. Invite supportive others to brainstorm with you on how to get things done. Working with a health coach on this can also be helpful. The reality is that much of your day-to-day pain is unpredictable, so seek out alternatives that encourage you to stay active or be productive in a relevant way.

Plan A-B-C-D-E may seem like just a mental trick, but if your pain stops you from doing what you set out to do that day, it can feel like an emotionally devastating defeat or failure. On the other hand, if you make a plan that allows for every possible physical state due to your pain, there is no failure — even if Plan D is to remain inactive or rest in bed. For your emotional state, and to live life as fully as possible, it's important to aim to accomplish at least *some* part of your adjustable plan. Avoid conceptu-alizing yourself as dysfunctional. Just because something cannot be done in one fashion, don't abandon it; instead, plan for reduced capacity. If you can't go for one long walk, break it into three short walks spaced at appropriate intervals. Plan your activities in accomplishable pieces for you. Don't give up the things that you enjoy.

> "Don't give up the things that you enjoy."

What we do in our lives in many ways defines us. It gives us a sense of meaning and purpose. There are many ways to demonstrate your value to yourself and others. You are not defined by any one set of tasks that you can — or can't — perform.

A client of mine, Tiana, once told me she couldn't be a grandmother because she couldn't lift and physically play with her grandchild. I asked her if those were the only ways she could interact with her grandchild. Was that the only way to be a grandmother? She understood. She substituted other activities for the highly physical play, sitting instead with her grandchild and playing non-physically demanding games. This brought her great joy.

Remember, if you can get something important done differently, or do something of equal value, you have salvaged an important part of your life.

Many people I've worked with are so angry at the limitations their pain causes them that they throw the baby out with the bathwater. For example, if they can't engage in their usual intimate activities with their partner, they may engage in none instead. Seek an alternate way. Different doesn't mean deficient.

If you can't go out to visit friends, invite them over. If you can't handle a physical visit, talk with them online. If a phone call is too much, text. The point is to never have to experience total physical defeat because of pain. And to never be without genuine expression of your life.

Embrace Cost-Benefit Living

When you live with chronic pain, any choice of physical activity may cost you in terms of increased pain and suffering. And you may feel it's worth it to be able to do those activities and get things done. But before you make the choice to try, also consider any downside to doing or not doing that activity. By this, I mean look at the emotional cost of either action or inaction, using a 0–10 scale (with 10 representing a very high, life-or-death kind or cost).

For example, say you want to mow the lawn, but you know that the exertion means you'll likely be laid up for days. Mowing the lawn might incur a 7 or an 8 in cost, because you might be more depressed and many other things may not get done. Then assess the cost of not mowing the lawn. You may be disappointed and troubled by your limitations; the job may not get done. These consequences may be a 4. Make your choice based upon a comparison of costs. Then, if you still want to choose the higher-priced activity, first look to see if you can reduce that cost. For instance, say you still want to mow the lawn, but maybe you can reduce the possibility of a flare-up by coming up with some creative approaches about how to get the job done with less strain.

It's important that you respect all of your needs when making these choices. You get to make your choices, you don't want to regret your decision. Cost-benefit assessments will help you avoid that.

Build a Pain Tolerance Bank Account

Each of us has only so much tolerance for pain and suffering. Before you choose to possibly bring more upon yourself, check your account. See if you can afford it.

You might assume your current tolerance is a fixed limit. It is not. Measure the choices you make to try to increase your tolerance over your current balance level. There are many approaches and strategies that can increase your pain tolerance and deepen your reserves — for example, yoga, aerobic exercise, cycling programs, meditation, breathing exercises, mental imagery, and biofeedback. Reducing depression, decreasing social isolation, and setting realistic expectations all help increase tolerance for pain. If you try out the approaches suggested here, you will find that the limits you have assumed are far from accurate.

Be mindful of your current tolerance levels even as they change. Everyone has their own experience and their own limits to how much they can bear. Avoid pushing your limits unnecessarily; instead, find ways to expand them safely. And call on professional guidance as you go.

Pace Yourself for Success

Be sure to pace yourself for success. In accordance with each activity, determine your best realistic pace, and pace yourself throughout the day.

Be aware that past habits and muscle memory may make this quite difficult. Especially if you're an athlete, dancer, martial artist, or high achiever, you may have great difficulty restraining yourself. You will be frustrated by setting a slower or less intense pace for yourself. But your current level of difficulty in a task is determined not by what you used to be able to do but by the physical state you're starting from now. Pace appropriate to today's reality.

If you are an athlete and you don't pace yourself around the physical reality you're starting from now, you're likely to reinjure yourself.

> **"Loss of function is more damaging than pain. Stay functional!"**

Whether you're an athlete or not, be sure to consult with a physical trainer or a physical therapist before you begin your activities, especially on good posture, form, and body mechanics. Practice these when engaging in all activities. Loss of function is more damaging than pain. Stay functional!

Credit yourself for making an equal effort today as before, even if, objectively, you're doing less than you could have in the past. If necessary, alternate heavier tasks with light tasks. Do the most difficult things when you're feeling most able to tolerate your efforts and be successful. Manage the time you spend to maximize the possibility of success; don't work through it unless you are likely to accomplish this.

Also pace yourself from day to day. Plan your weeks around getting things done, even if slowly, and remaining at a higher level of functioning. Use time management skills to help you accomplish this. Be realistic when assigning time frames to finish things. Don't try to do too much at once; instead, make your activities accomplishable.

You can strategize to make accomplishing tasks easier. Review your weekly tasks and eliminate the ones that are not necessary. Make a schedule for each day either the night before or first thing in the morning. Think about what each task involves in terms of the amount of time and effort it requires. You can also include rest breaks in your daily plan; combine chores and errands so you can get more done with less effort; and organize work areas so you can get more done with less energy.

In other words, you want to redesign how you go about things in ways that require less effort and time. Consider task- and time-management techniques to aid you in this. For example, if extended sitting to read is too painful, study speed reading or try reading while quietly strolling around the room. If your memory is challenged by your pain, study mnemonics (improving memory techniques). Use advanced preparation and assembly-line approaches to household tasks like cooking and doing laundry. This approach has been consistently reported to be helpful by all my clients who have tried it. You can also delegate tasks, to conserve energy.

When planning for self-care and other activities, aim to understand energy conservation. Coping with pain during activity requires physical, emotional, and psychological energy. You may not be mindful of how much energy you have available at any moment or how much energy you will have to spend to do something. Over time, you can track this, as well as enhance it through energy-building activities such as getting moving, doing some cardio, playing some music, reducing stress, avoiding caffeine, drinking less alcohol, staying hydrated, eating energizing foods (fish, bananas, brown rice, sweet potatoes, eggs, apples, berries, dark chocolate), getting a massage, or completing something challenging. Don't allow your pain to drain you. Counter it with positive, energizing life experiences.

> "Ask for help when you need it. Receiving love and support from others will enhance your ability to function and reduce isolation."

Equally important, try not to resist engaging the aid of others. Remember that limits to your functioning are not just de-energizing physically but also challenging emotionally. Counter the emotional toll with positive emotional connectivity. Ask for help and inspiration when you need it — from family, friends, and co-workers. Receiving love and support from others will not only enhance your ability to function, it will also offset your sense of isolation, reducing the drain of emotional suffering.

Balance Rest and Activity

Learn your body's signs of getting tired. Become aware of the difference between physical and emotional fatigue. At these moments, determine whether rest, relaxation, or emotional support is what's most needed. Take breaks during or between tasks to conserve your energy. Or proactively add energizing moments — such as stretching, a brief meditation, or a breathing exercise — in between other activities to help keep your energy from lagging. Get enough sleep. (You can use the approaches outlined in chapter 5, "Sleep Disruption," to help keep your energy up.) And get into the habit of listening to your body. For example, if you feel tired after lunch every day, take a rest break or brief nap.

Manage Flare-Ups Proactively

The traditional treatment model does not consider what happens existentially when you experience a pain flare-up. Flare-ups frighten and traumatize you over time. They undermine your sense of safety and recovery, both in the moment and looking into the future. So we can predict that when you have a flare-up, it will produce stress, anger, frustration, negative thoughts, anxiety, and feelings of helplessness and discouragement in addition to physical suffering.

If you plan for these impacts with a physical flare-up plan, you can feel reassured that you have techniques to help reduce your pain. If your flare-up plan lessens your fears about what the increased pain means for the present and in the future, it will reduce your stress.

Planning is crucial to recovery. When your chronic pain is more active, use flare-up management techniques to lessen the pain before and after engaging in tasks. Analyze your flare-up patterns. Find the physical and emotional triggers for your flare-ups. Keep a written record. Develop a flare-up plan for dealing with increased pain and dysfunction. For instance, you might take longer and more frequent rest breaks if it enables you to accomplish more.

> "Have a plan for emotional support and back-up."

Then use what you've learned about lessening your pain in a more formal and organized manner. Your flare-up plan should be based on your experience with methods and treatments that have already demonstrated they can help with your pain. When you have a flare-up, you'll want to know exactly how you can respond to it in a stepwise, integrated fashion based on an analysis of past successes. Organize the steps such that one supports the other. For example, what to do first? Lying down, using ice or heat, stretching, medication, rest, exercise, meditation, massage, or physical therapy? In what combination? Aim to have a planned, orderly counter to flare-ups prepared, something self-supportive and constructive, based on data from past experience. You are constantly gaining the knowledge and experience to be able to figure out the optimal approach.

Also develop an emotional flare-up plan to help deal with the emotional impact of a pain relapse. Have no doubt: Renewed pain can be traumatic. Review what you have experienced when this happens, and have a plan for emotional support and backup. When you know in advance what you will do, flare-ups will be much less stressful emotionally and will create significantly less pain and trauma.

These plans are similar to the advance plans people use in case of relapse of substance abuse so they know exactly what to do (call a sponsor and attend more meetings).

Work in Partnership

Include your health care providers, family, and friends in your recovery. Having others to brainstorm with and to help you achieve your goals is essential, especially given the challenges and unpredictable occurrences in chronic pain. You can prevent loss of function by always having some way to get things done even if you can't do it all by yourself. Seek to accomplish your tasks by getting help from others when you need it. Help them to know what would be meaningful to you and doable for them. If you do, your friends and family will feel they are contributing something of value, and you will receive more emotional support as well. This will also help prevent friends and family from becoming resentful, tired, unempathetic, or avoidant and experiencing helper burnout.

Let go of the notion that people will think less of you if you ask for help. Quite the contrary — friends and relatives usually feel helpless to help you manage your pain. Letting them help will be a gift to them as well as to you.

Practice Supportive Techniques

Practices such as proper breathing, positive affirmations, and personal validation will also help support you while performing tasks and in between.

In addition, don't hesitate to try self-help or labor-saving devices. Tools and prosthetics make the impossible possible and are there to help you maintain your function, not stigmatize you; if you accept your devices, others will. Consider the example of Stephen Hawking, the world's leading physicist, who can speak only with the aid of a computer.

Chapter 7

Physical De-Conditioning

The damage chronic pain causes to your physical state and functioning can disrupt and change many of your physical behaviors and, ultimately, your capacity. Yet these changes are frequently minimized or overlooked. I have seen over time that when these relationships — between chronic pain, physical activity and conditioning, and level of functioning — are neglected, pain treatments and interventions often fail. Understanding these relationships can be critical to your recovery.

In this chapter, we look at an additional, highly significant spectrum of physical collateral damages that can result from chronic pain — from atrophy, energy loss, damage to physical systems, and complications from medication to changes in pain-tolerance levels and body weight. If you notice stress or tension arising as you read, remember that acknowledging negative realities is the first step toward empowerment. The next step is to learn about the many ways to minimize or eliminate the power of these impacts through the strategies in the Recovery section. Once recovery strategies are understood, you can move toward flourishing and growth.

ATROPHY

Chapter 6 described physical impacts such as avoidance of ordinary movement and use of guarding and protecting behaviors. These impacts can eventually lead to additional negative outcomes, including increasing physical weakness, loss of flexibility and strength, loss of overall physical conditioning, and even physical atrophy, defined as the wasting away or reduction in size of parts of the body. These losses, which often grow over the time that you are limited physically, undercut structural support to the injured area of your body and result in a decrease in function. By the reports of many hundreds of clients over the last twenty years, I've found that physical de-conditioning can contribute up to 30 percent more pain and significantly affect your body's ability to recover.

De-conditioning involves muscle breakdown, loss of muscle strength and elasticity, and weaker supportive structures in many areas of the body. De-conditioned muscles can result in impaired motor control, poorer balance and mobility, increased body fat, and even osteoporosis and obesity. Prolonged de-conditioning can also lead to atrophy of muscles and bones, with a loss of mass, size, and strength. However, given enough time and effort, this type of atrophy can usually be reversed with exercise.

Let's take the case of back pain. The greater your core, lower back, and abdominal strength, the more you can support damaged areas and alleviate your pain. That's why core strengthening is the central focus in much physical therapy. It's why my clients who find their way back to some level of good physical conditioning also have less pain and a higher level of physical functioning.

Ultimately, de-conditioning can also weaken the immune system and undermine your body's ability to heal from injury. Decreased conditioning and atrophy can hamper your body's ability to heal from blood clots; it can cause shallow breathing and suppressed coughing that raise the risk of pneumonia. It can lead to a host of problems, including sodium and water retention in the kidneys; raised heart rate, blood pressure, and metabolic rate; decreased cardiovascular capacity; impaired gastrointestinal functioning; hormonal imbalances; difficulty sleeping; and loss of appetite. The potential impact on your levels of pain from these complications is obvious. But the reverse is also true: Regaining at least some extent of physical conditioning is almost always possible. By pursuing reconditioning, many of my clients experience less pain, strengthen their immune systems, and increase their overall functioning.

ENERGY LOSS

Dealing with chronic pain requires energy; it's an energy conservation-and-building task. This means you must learn to manage your physical and emotional energy—both of which are limited resources. Anything that drains your physical or emotional energy limits your ability to contend with and manage your pain.

Energy loss thus affects your potential to maintain overall functioning.

It's easy to get into a vicious cycle with energy loss. The physical and emotional energy you spend dealing with loss of function can make you feel fatigued. Reduced energy, in turn, means less power to function, which increases stress — and therefore pain.

> "You have far more power to build energy than you suspect, despite the impacts of your pain."

Loss of energy undermines your quality of life, reducing motivation and diminishing your ability to perform tasks and cope with stressors. De-conditioning and inflammation may cause loss of energy. The same may happen if you experience a flare-up of pain.

Chronic pain may be associated with anemia, a problem in the blood. Overextending yourself, or difficulty in pacing yourself, can reduce your energy. It may be hard to know when you've reached your limit.

Your surroundings may also add to your fatigue. For example, a person with arthritis may have difficulty dealing with uncomfortable furniture and lots of stairs. Loud noises and warmer temperatures may be tiring for some.

In chronic pain, there are many threats to your needs, both present and future. These threats often produce not only anxiety and anger but feelings of helplessness, hopelessness, and depression, which cause a further loss of energy. Negative emotional states have the potential to create reactions that fatigue the adrenal glands. Excessive or unresolved negative emotions generate chronic stress, which in turn saps energy. Adrenal exhaustion from severe chronic pain and stress leaves one in an ongoing state of fatigue.

If you become more aware of what contributes to your energy loss, you will be better able to offset it. The Recovery section in this chapter will reassure you that you are not helpless to deal with energy loss. In fact, you have far more power and agency to build energy than you suspect, despite the impacts of your pain.

Chronic pain can be made worse by existing medical conditions, and it can also make them worse. Atrophy, loss of energy, and other challenges enumerated here can snowball across increasing periods of pain and lead to damage to physical systems. For example, chronic pain may contribute to the development of hyper- or hypoglycemia, pituitary–adrenal problems, and weight loss or gain. It may decrease the body's production of natural painkillers or weaken your immune system. It can contribute to the onset of low blood sugar, asthma and other breathing problems, skin disorders, hormonal imbalances, and menstrual problems. It may increase your risk of diabetes and heart disease.

Meanwhile, existing medical conditions — including obesity, headaches, hypertension, lupus, osteoporosis, tooth decay, attention deficit, herpes, and depression or other mental health conditions — can complicate or increase chronic pain. This possibility is something to be aware of and to try to prevent or counter. If these conditions are worsened by your pain, they can further undermine your functioning and your ability to recover.

DAMAGE FROM MEDICATION

Collateral damages from chronic pain may also arise, ironically, from efforts to treat it — specifically, from the many medications that can be prescribed in an effort to help. Your medications may be necessary for you to have less pain, but they may also have a negative impact on your physical state or overall functioning, which will then add to your pain problem. People with chronic pain often face this choice: What is more important to you, less pain or higher functioning? Most of my clients prefer higher functioning.

Unfortunately, you may not know the scope and extent of the negative consequences you are incurring from your pain medications.

To illustrate this, consider narcotic medications, which work by binding to receptors in the brain to block the feeling of pain. These drugs impair attention, concentration, memory, energy, and decision-making — all critical to your ability to function. They can also cause negative behaviors, even personality changes, and can mask depression and suppress other emotions designed to help you. Narcotic medications are also addictive and often counterproductive. The problem is, the pills are a passive approach, and not rehabilitative or curative. They may make you more lethargic and encourage you to be less physical They may discourage you from using more active and *physically* rehabilitative recovery-based practices and from active use of your skills and innate potential. Why do any of these things when you can take a pill?

Other types of pain medication also have negative side effects, which can add to loss of physical conditioning. For example, common side effects of muscle relaxants include drowsiness, confusion, nausea, and vomiting. Side effects from anticonvulsant medications include weight gain or loss, upset stomach, loss of appetite, skin rashes, drowsiness or confusion, and headaches. Common side effects of antidepressants include dry mouth, constipation, blurred vision, weight gain, sleepiness, problems urinating, and sexual problems. Less commonly, these drugs can also have damaging effects on the heart and lungs.

Nerve-pain medications such as gabapentin and Lyrica (pregabalin), while helpful in relieving pain, can also cause significant problems with concentration, attention, and short-term memory, and are quite sedating; and longer-term impact on functioning can also occur.

Excessive use of Tylenol (acetaminophen) can cause severe damage to your liver. Nonsteroidal anti-inflammatory drugs (NSAIDs) and acetaminophen in high doses, or taken for a long time, can cause stomach ulcers and bleeding and liver or kidney damage. Any of these drugs may also interact with other medicines or make certain medical conditions worse.

Like all the physical impacts we have reviewed so far, the first step toward recovery is becoming aware of what your own collateral damages are. Once you do that, and recognize their importance, you'll be more highly motivated to counter them. This can best be done by finding rehabilitation-based approaches that, unlike medications, don't have side effects that decrease functioning. Many of these approaches are covered in this chapter's Recovery section.

CHANGED PAIN THRESHOLDS

Your tolerance for pain can either help reduce suffering and dysfunction or increase it. It is important to be fully aware of and attend to your pain, and not block or numb it in a way that increases risk, as there are many variables that can increase your pain beyond what would be expected with your injury.

Your individual sensitivity to pain is governed by a complex interaction of genes, cognitions, mood, environment, situation, and day-to-day experiences as well as early-life experiences. Think about how your caretakers tolerated and expressed pain. How did they respond to yours? Families develop a specific style of dealing with pain that includes the thoughts and emotional responses that accompany pain. Your level of tolerance and resistance to pain may have been learned by observing and imitating their behavior in response to pain, or by how they reacted to you.

In addition, all the physical impacts described so far will eventually affect your ability to tolerate pain. If you suffer from chronic pain, you likely already keep pain in your awareness beyond what is necessary for safety. This happens when you don't know whether your pain signals discomfort or danger. When you do this, however, you are putting your nervous system on heightened alert, a setting that amplifies pain and lowers your pain tolerance.

Factors that contribute to heightened alert include repetitive unexplained pain, treatment failure, the passage of time, physical weakness, negative judgmental thoughts, negative emotions, and chronic stress. Fear of pain and reinjury, fear of activity and rehabilitation, excessive pain attention, and pain catastrophizing can all lower pain tolerance, thus increasing your subjective experience of the pain.

Some conditions and medications can also decrease pain tolerance in problematic ways, such as when opioid medications cause a condition called opioid-induced hyperalgesia. This is caused by opioid consumption over time, which in many cases can alter brain chemistry in a way that creates lower pain tolerance.

WEIGHT CHANGES

There's a clear link between being beyond the recommended healthy weight for you and having chronic pain. With chronic pain, the extra weight may make it harder to recover. Weight loss can weaken you physically, as well as potentially undermine your immune system. Weight gain can add more pain and disability.

This is understandable considering the strain that extra weight places on the body. If you were carrying a thirty- to forty-pound pack on your back, even with a healthy body you'd notice the weight and start feeling pain after just an hour or two. The problem isn't only mechanical, however. Being overweight can also place a strain on the body's circulatory system, which in turn can lead to inflammation in the joints and severe, chronic headaches.

Inactivity, loss of physical conditioning, depression, stress, and medication are the primary contributors to weight gain among people with chronic pain. People's eating patterns are often keyed into their regular activity and exercise levels. This can be seen among athletes, who often gain substantial weight after retirement. Same eating, but less activity and exercise. For many people with chronic pain, food can be part of a negative self-medication regimen that results in depression- or stress-induced overeating and poor diet. This may also be true of alcohol consumption, which in turn can contribute to weight gain.

Certain antidepressants, corticosteroids, lithium, tranquilizers, phenothiazine, and drugs that increase fluid retention can cause weight gain. People taking opioid medications often gain weight; opioids cause a "sugar desire effect" on opioid receptors that leads to a preference for sweet foods. Weight gain on opioids can be profound, with some people doubling their weight within a few years. Opioid use may also cause blood sugar levels to be very unstable and may cause hypoglycemia. Consequently, the combination of severe chronic pain and opioid treatment can cause a condition called deranged glucose metabolism, which includes a potent desire to eat primarily sugars and starches, often with little protein or fat intake. Note that diet itself can contribute to inflammation and thus undermine the immune system, inhibiting recovery. Both dietary changes and weight changes can affect people's willingness to try or stick with a therapy, jeopardizing their recovery.

RECOVERY: PHYSICAL RE-CONDITIONING

You may be in a situation where ordinary movement is severely challenged by pain or by anxiety about reinjury. If so, the notion of becoming physically re-conditioned may be daunting indeed. Any exercise could cause substantial pain flare-ups and new fears. This is often the case when you are first injured, but it can also continue when pain becomes chronic.

Nonetheless, overcoming the challenges and moving toward re-conditioning is one of the biggest steps you can take toward your own recovery. To counter physical de-conditioning, you need to reconceptualize what's required for physical recovery. The nine strategies covered here fall into two overarching categories: minimizing loss of your current physical conditioning, and restoring or enhancing your general physical conditioning.

> "Reconceptualize what's required for physical recovery."

Minimize Loss of Physical Conditioning

Physical de-activation begins the de-conditioning process and tends to be initially supported by advice from providers. For example, to not do "things that cause pain." Staying inactive may bring considerable relief from your pain and quiet your fears of reinjury. So, you may ask, how is it possible to maintain physical conditioning or minimize de-conditioning under these circumstances?

First, realize that you need not take an all-or-nothing approach. Perhaps you believe that because you cannot do some things physically, you cannot do *anything*. You may believe that your pain and structural issues prevent you from doing anything that might positively affect your level of physical conditioning. Know, instead, that there is always something you can do within your own capacities.

Seek Opportunities

Exercising with chronic pain is quite different from ordinary exercise. If you were a regular exerciser or athlete, you likely know that pain doesn't always mean harm. For example, muscles can ache after weightlifting, especially when you're in the process of building them up.

In chronic pain, the relationship between pain and harm is often much less clearly defined, despite your providers' best efforts to inform you. You are not alone in not understanding what causes you pain, or in not knowing whether your pain indicates danger of increased pain, harm, or reinjury. This uncertainty often results from an information or communication breakdown with providers. (You'll find more about working with your providers in chapter 18, "Mastering the Treatment Experience.")

> **"Take your focus off what you can't do and on to what is possible."**

As we discussed in a previous chapter, one way to challenge inactivity is by viewing everyday life as an athletic event, where all physical movement offers the possibility for exercise. In the movie *The Karate Kid*, much was made of the training the sensei used with his student. He used ordinary activities, like painting a fence and waxing a car, to provide his student with physical conditioning and martial arts training. You also can look for opportunities to preserve or enhance conditioning where you can find them in your daily actions. For example, in opening a door, walking, getting out of bed or up from a chair, standing and sitting, or getting dressed. Take your focus *off* what you can't do and *on* to what is possible.

Investigate Safe Movement

In addition to learning to think like an athlete, you can investigate and apply the lessons on risk assessment outlined in the Recovery section of chapter 6. As an intelligent person, you're not about to do something that hurts without assessing whether it is causing you harm. So, before attempting to condition or re-condition, you must address the most significant barriers to safely moving forward.

Make your best efforts to get the information you need to approach physical re-conditioning safely. You need to understand the structural mechanisms that generate your pain, how activity affects them, and when to be concerned about exacerbation or reinjury. In my practice, I often help clients with this investigation. However, much of this information can be obtained with an organized approach to questioning your providers, such as using the following questions with all your providers:

- What is the exact anatomical/structural explanation for my pain condition?
- Why do my structural problems cause specific pain in each specific area?
- Are there factors besides my structural issues that contribute to or cause any of my symptoms (such as de-activation, de-conditioning, posture, guarding and protecting, pain attention, medication, treatment side effects)?
- How will particular activities affect my pain? (Ask specifically in terms of activities important to you.) Do I need to stop, or can I modify these activities?
- How long will I be in pain? (Ask for statistics.)
- How long will my pain impact my functioning and how much?
- What is the most likely course of my recovery? What benchmarks should I expect to see? Can I eventually resume my regular activities? (Again, ask specifically about important activities.)
- Can I achieve my ultimate physical goals? (Ask specifically about your important goals.)
- How specifically are my treatments likely to help my pain problem? What are the likely side effects? What impact will my treatment have on pain reduction, range of motion, functioning?
- Am I safe to engage in activities? (Again, ask specifically about your most important activities.) What are the worst-case scenarios for reinjury or additional injury from rehabilitation exercises and other activities?

You will also need a documented record of your pain experience. There are apps that can help you document your pain, functional levels, flare-ups, side effects, changes, and treatment outcomes across time. Using your providers' answers plus your record can produce greater clarity on the safety issue, for both you and your providers. (These approaches are explained in greater detail in chapters 17 and 18.) They will help you understand whether there is actual risk of reinjury, and what it would take for that to happen.

All in all, understanding how to move safely will help you re-condition and reverse atrophy, boost energy, and improve damaged physical systems.

Use Professionals

To see where you are in this process, you and your providers will need to work together to assess your starting point. This work will be based on shared attention to your records, documentation of your past and current pain, and your present state of recovery. Ask direct questions of your providers: Do I need occupational therapy to keep me active in ordinary physical activities? Do I need rehabilitation, working with a physical therapist? Or do I need physical re-conditioning, working with a physical trainer who specializes in chronic pain?

Chronic pain can de-activate you rapidly, so simply getting moving again in basic ways is an important first step. When activities like physical therapy are undertaken prematurely, before someone's genuine need for physical re-activation has been met, it often fails. In such cases, some folks draw the erroneous conclusion that physical therapy is unhelpful, when in truth, they simply weren't ready for that level of treatment — they were out of shape for rehabilitation. They needed to activate and reactivate in more basic ways first.

Physical re-conditioning at any significant level should occur after reactivation and rehabilitation, to consolidate and strengthen the gains those have brought.

No matter where you are in this continuum, work with your providers to develop a time-limited, stepwise, overall reactivation, rehabilitation, and re-conditioning plan. You need a plan with clear goals, clearly defined objectives, benchmarks, and timelines. This can be even more challenging if you were never interested in exercise or physical conditioning before. What's in it for you? This may be an important step in your journey of personal transformation.

One approach I suggest is to imagine your own ideal body fitness level. For example, would you like to achieve all-around good physical conditioning or something more ambitious — like that of a swimmer, runner, gymnast, martial artist, or mountain climber? This decision helps you set goals and measure outcomes. Consult with a doctor, physical therapist, or physical trainer for routines and plans for how to achieve your goals and assess if they are realistic.

The most powerful motivation for this can be found as you experience how physical conditioning can reduce your pain, promote healing, and make it less likely you'll experience a flare-up or reinjury. Good conditioning through exercise will also increase your sense of well-being. It will result in overall reduced stress and increased energy. Conditioning through exercise is your best insurance for maintaining physical stability and continuing to improve in your recovery.

There are many ways to exercise even with chronic pain. Remember — you are living life as an athletic event! There is no physical action you cannot turn into an exercise or that can't be easily converted to some form of strengthening and/or stretching. These actions may not be the equivalent of a serious physical training program, but they are vital steps toward counteracting physical decline.

> "There is no physical action you cannot turn into an exercise or that can't be easily converted to some form of strengthening and/or stretching."

When you are ready to engage in a more serious program of physical conditioning, seek out the advice and support of all relevant providers. Together, reassess your current pain and recovery state. With this information in hand, commit to strengthening all the areas of your body you can. Work with physical trainers experienced in helping people with chronic pain to develop your approach and goals. I have sent many of my clients to such providers with consistent progress and success. I watched as these people attained a superior level of conditioning — even in some cases beyond their pre-injury condition — all with no instances of reinjury.

There are many terrific results of an increase in physical conditioning to look forward to. Usually, people experience a comprehensive improvement in function. They develop reinjury resistance. Their energy is substantially restored. And their pain is reduced.

Exercise Appropriately

The following tips are based on my experience with clients undergoing a conditioning program.

Once you have your plan for conditioning in place, look for ways to integrate exercise into your daily schedule and routine in addition to your formal workouts. Make exercise central to your life, and high on your priority list.

Most conditioning programs will focus on core stabilization and strengthening the pelvis, back, abdomen, and chest. Core strengthening improves posture, balance, strength, endurance, and coordination.

Exercise is usually enhanced by learning proper breathing techniques to assist you in both activity and pain control. Also, to help you avoid strain or reinjury, pay attention to the state of tension in your muscles when you exercise. If possible, practice relaxation, meditation, and biofeedback as part of your activities. Consider if Pilates, yoga, tai chi, or qigong should be part of your plan.

Make sure your program considers the physical mechanisms of your pain, so that you can gear your activities in ways less likely to provoke muscle spasms. Avoid exercises that can cause inflammation of your chronic structural issues.

Make sure your program adjusts for and corrects compensatory physical behaviors (guarding and protecting behaviors) if at all possible. When exercising, try to reduce attention to your pain by communicating any concerns you have to your trainer and getting adequate information to feel reassured about safety.

Follow a Progressive Program

For all activities, plan for increasing levels of difficulty to move toward higher levels of energy, physical capacity, and functioning. Be specific in timelines and benchmarks for this. Monitor improvements in flexibility, strength, range of motion, and level of functioning and activity, as well as reduced pain.

As you proceed, be prepared to modify or transform activities and tasks as needed. Always have a back-up plan, so that there's always something you can do. If that is impossible — and it may be at times — plan to congratulate yourself for your effort and intention. *There is no failure here.*

Get a Medication Assessment

The Recovery sections are full of examples of alternatives to pain medication. The more of these approaches you apply, the less of a need you will have for medications. The most important consideration, of course, beyond discomfort and dangerous side effects, is the impact of many medications on functioning.

There are times when medication is the only option for managing chronic pain. However, overall, too much emphasis and reliance are placed on drugs — and too little attention is given to drugs' impact on functioning. Remember, chronic pain is much more than just your injury. Much of the collateral damage that occurs is the result of how your pain impacts your ability to function. Isn't it? Pain relief is obviously your first desire. But if the price of relief is the diminishment of your life, is it worth it?

Be sure to measure the price you pay for your medication's pain relief against its cost to your ability to participate in your life.

Be willing to investigate the promises and possibilities of alternative treatments and practices, such as naturopathy, meditation, acupuncture, yoga, exercise, diet, and especially stress and pain management counseling. (You'll find more information about the benefits of counseling and stress management in chapter 8, "Cognitive Impacts.")

Optimize Your Weight

There are myriad approaches to optimizing weight, whether that includes weight loss or weight gain. Be sure to consult with your physician, and possibly a weight loss program, naturopath, and/or nutritionist, to help you with this.

Many people with chronic pain gain a substantial amount of weight, in many cases fifty to one hundred pounds. And there are many reasons why people with chronic pain

> "It's easier to lose weight if you try not to lose the entertainment and pleasure value that food gives you."

may have difficulty losing weight, including lifelong habits, difficulty exercising and being active, and a sense of already feeling deprived of many pleasurable things. Based on my experience with many clients facing this challenge, here are some recommendations.

First, assess all the reasons why it will be hard for you to lose weight.

Then, be honest with yourself about what is at stake. For instance, I've had hundreds of clients who can't have a needed surgery, or can't do the physical therapy they need, unless they lose weight. This puts them at risk not just for the downward spiral that chronic pain can become but for survival itself. Fighting weight loss may be a fight for your life. And losing weight may be the very thing that can move you toward reclaiming your life.

To lose weight often requires you to transform how you think about food and eating. Be thoughtful in your choice of and preparation of food. Always remember, it's easier to lose weight if your diet doesn't deprive you. Try not to lose the entertainment and pleasure value that food gives you. Choose healthy alternatives and be creative in your cooking. There are many available alternatives to your current diet that can help you retain the pleasure in what you eat.

Improve Your Pain Thresholds

Everyone's life experiences and adaptions to challenges are unique; so are the ways each person has learned to feel and deal with pain. Perception of pain in terms of its discomfort and negative qualities can vary tremendously among individuals. This perception often determines how much pain affects physical, emotional, and psychological functioning. Pain is also a cumulative experience. Your personal pain tolerance may be reduced (made more limited) by things like experiencing pain repeatedly, having a fear of this repetition, and by the extent of the impact on your functioning.

When defining your own pain tolerance, understand these two things: It's subjective, and it fluctuates. Also remember that the amount of atten-

> **"Feeling safer leads to higher pain tolerance."**

tion you apply to your pain is, to a large extent, voluntary. There are many examples of people who "adapt" to pain and become more resistant to its unpleasantness and impacts. Soldiers, police officers, football players and other athletes, and martial artists, among others. Therefore, we know it's possible to lower or raise your pain threshold and decrease or increase your pain tolerance over time. Generally, this can be accomplished through the information-seeking and risk-assessment strategies discussed previously.

In-depth knowledge of the physical danger your pain represents also can increase your pain tolerance. Pain from conditions like tinnitus, ordinary headaches, a stubbed toe, or even a simple broken arm are easier to tolerate because we know the extent of the danger. Physical injury that is known and curable is more tolerable. In chronic pain conditions, this level of exactness is often lacking. This leaves most people with increased anxiety and a lower pain tolerance.

Chapter 18, "Mastering the Treatment Experience," outlines a "composite approach" to preparing for health care visits and then tracking and comparing provider responses to your questions. Using this approach, you can get closer to a true understanding of your actual condition and your level of safety. Feeling safer leads to higher pain tolerance.

There are also many myths about how to increase pain tolerance. For example, here's one myth that has persisted since Rocky first ran up the steps of the Philadelphia Museum of Art: Repeated exposure to pain increases pain tolerance. This myth is false. In fact, it's often just the opposite: Repeated exposure to pain can cause an area to have increased sensitivity to pain.

So here are some of the most successful, long-proven techniques for increasing pain tolerance:

Meditative and/or Zen breathing exercises, such as those used in yoga, meditation, and martial arts, can be quite effective. They typically involve slow, deep, measured breathing. In almost all cases, this breathing has been shown to successfully reduce pain, related anxiety, and stress, and elevate pain tolerance levels. A common example is the use of breathing techniques during childbirth to increase tolerance to sharp, stabbing pains.

Meditation, a practice that includes helpful breathing techniques, has been shown to be effective at increasing tolerance for pain in the short term — and for extended periods. Meditation appears to be particularly effective in managing chronic pain. Many of my clients have benefited from meditation sessions with a marked reduction in pain perception. Mindfulness meditation is one form that has well-documented benefits.

Accurate self-talk has also been shown to increase pain tolerance during episodes of acute pain. For instance, athletes who were given balanced and nuanced coaching statements to internalize during training sessions were found better able to cope with pain than those who dwelled only on the negative aspects of their pain. Perhaps you have said to yourself during a pain flare-up, "My pain is killing me! I'll always be in pain!" Now imagine saying instead, "My pain is really unpleasant and hard to handle. But I know many ways to deal with it. I don't really know if I'll always have pain, but I do know I'll do my best to deal with it." Accurate self-talk can often generate at least short-term benefits to pain tolerance, whereas negative, inaccurate self-talk is likely to increase both your stress and your pain.

Stress-management techniques for chronic pain use several cognitive and behavioral techniques that will be discussed in more detail in later chapters. It is a given that stress increases pain and makes it harder to resist. This can be altered substantially by self-explo-ration in counseling and by learning various stress-management techniques (including emotion regulation, which is discussed in chapter 16, "Mental Health Impacts and Risk Factors.") Handling stress is an extremely important aspect of pain tolerance — and overall recovery and thriving.

Remember, there are two pains in chronic pain: the physical injury and the emotional and psychological pain caused by chronic pain that affects your life. Reducing your stress and learning to manage it more successfully can reduce both physical and emotional pain.

Chapter 8

Cognitive Impacts

Pain is distracting and disruptive not to just physical action but to mental action as well. A number of my clients have borne witness to this. They find that their ability to think clearly, concentrate, pay attention, focus, remember things, and make decisions is challenged by the multiple impacts caused by their pain. I had one client who was trying to prepare for the bar exam but couldn't retain enough information, or successfully focus and concentrate on what he was studying, to complete the exam and become an attorney. Clients of mine who go back to school to seek a new occupation less impacted by their pain often find that cognitive alterations interfere with learning new information and participating in class. In fact, people with chronic pain can find it challenging just to stay on top of ordinary tasks and be organized and structured in their day-to-day tasks. Pain can actually rewire the brain in ways that affect its overall structure and function.

Alterations in cognitive functioning can eat away at your self-esteem, not just your cognitive skills. Your speed and ability to respond to cognitive tasks, including executing and completing structured tasks, may be affected. It may become more difficult to process multiple things at once and to react to ongoing changes in your environment. You may become less competent at emotional decision-making. Loss of cognitive functioning may also include negative impact on motor performance.

Cognitive impairments can be caused by physical collateral damage from your pain as well as some pain treatments that can affect your brain structure and chemistry. Too much pain can even interfere with learning all the things you need to learn to help you counter the consequences of your pain.

DIMINISHED EXECUTIVE FUNCTIONING

Over time you may experience impairment in any of these ways:

- Loss of focus (attention, concentration)
- Difficulties with memory (short-term memory)
- Impaired mental agility (mental flexibility, verbal ability, and processing speed)

The above cognitive abilities are part of your *executive functioning*, which is a term for the part of the brain's processes related to planning, managing multiple tasks, and self-regulating emotionally. As has been said about many things, including cognition: If you don't use it, you lose it.

Cognitive dysfunction can add to your overall loss of function, increase suffering, and increase your pain through the stress it creates.

RECOVERY: REMEDIATION WITH MIND-BODY SUPPORT

While the cognitive impact of chronic pain can be devastating, the good news is there are ways to minimize or even eliminate the impacts. This, in part, is thanks to something called neuroplasticity. Neuroplasticity is a concept that explains how the brain can change in response to training and experience.

The sections below outline seven approaches to help maintain or restore your cognitive functioning. These approaches have been used successfully by a number of my clients, and are also being used to help patients with brain injuries, attention deficits, and other cognitive challenges.

Use Cognitive Remediation Therapy

Two techniques used to offset cognitive impacts include cognitive remediation and counseling. Cognitive remediation therapy has been used for traumatic brain injury, attention deficit, schizophrenia, and other conditions where cognitive skills are compromised. This set of techniques is designed to preserve and enhance "thinking skills" and can be thought of as a form of cognitive rehabilitation — exercise for the brain. Cognitive remediation is a mental workout designed to strengthen or enhance brain function and cognition. It involves training in a set of tasks specifically designed to improve cognitive abilities. The domains that are targeted depend on your need but can include any cognitive function. The expected result is a direct positive impact on preventing, stabilizing, and/or eliminating cognitive deficits. Cognitive remediation therapy techniques can be delivered via computerized programs of varying length and complexity or can be undertaken one-on-one with a trained clinician.

Nearly every cognitive remediation approach makes use of *strategic* and/or *drill and practice* techniques. Drill and practice consists of practicing a problem or exercise until a peak level of performance is reached. This is done by training the brain functions with exercises that are regularly repeated. Strategic training helps you learn strategies for solving cognitive problems and enhancing performance, such as the use of memory. For example, you may practice memorizing a shopping list by using a mental image composed of the various ingredients.

Use Counseling

Cognitive therapies can help address the impact of undermined cognitive function, as well as support recovery. Trained counselors can help people cope with cognitive impairment by teaching compensatory strategies, providing support, and helping them deal with feelings about their cognitive issues. Close members of a person's family are sometimes included in at least some therapy sessions. This can help family members prepare for and cope with the changes that cognitive impairment may bring about in their loved one and the effects these changes may have on daily life. All these approaches are useful in understanding, counteracting, and even preventing cognitive decline.

Learn Mind-Body Techniques

Mind-body techniques are practices that strengthen the connection between a person's emotional, psychological, and physical aspects. Examples include breathing techniques, guided mental imagery, progressive muscle relaxation techniques, yoga, and tai chi. These practices include developing mental focus, controlled breathing, and body movements to help relax the body and the mind. They can also be used to control pain, stress, anxiety, and depression. They are very useful for overall health.

Sarah was a client of mine who had been through multiple back surgeries. She had significant chronic pain despite many medical interventions, including medication to help her reduce her pain and its impacts. She began the practice of tai chi and mindfulness meditation, and over time she mastered them. As a result, she was able to reduce her overall pain and disruption of her cognitive functioning by up to 30 percent. She also gained a greater appreciation of her own innate ability to affect the impacts of her chronic pain.

Most mind-body techniques have the opposite effect on the brain as chronic pain: They *enhance* cognitive functioning rather than degrade it. Mind-body practices seem to exert a protective effect on brain functioning and can counteract the cognitive problems caused by chronic pain.

> **"When you change your mindset, you can change your brain."**

It is important to note that the mind is not the same as the brain. The mind consists of mental states such as thoughts, emotions, beliefs, attitudes, and images. The brain is the hardware that allows us to experience those mental states. Balancing your mind, your emotions, and your physicality will help you feel more centered and mentally focused. Keep in mind this important point: When you change your mindset, you can change your brain.

Get Moving

When you exercise, blood flow increases and your brain is exposed to more oxygen and nutrients. This induces the release of beneficial proteins in the brain that are nourishing and help keep your brain cells healthy as well as promote the growth of new neurons. Neurons are the building blocks of the brain. This is why physical activity and exercise are consistently found to not only prevent cognitive decline but help to restore cognitive functioning. Individuals who are physically active are much less likely to experience cognitive decline. So physical activity can serve as a counter and preventive to the cognitive impacts of chronic pain. I have observed this in all of my clients as they engaged in physical reactivation, exercise, and reconditioning.

Exercise can also help boost thinking processes and memory indirectly by improving your mood and your sleep and reducing stress, depression, and anxiety. Less stress means less interference with cognitive functioning.

Therefore, make physical activity and exercise a priority. All activity helps. For example, walking, doing dishes, cooking, thirty minutes on an exercise bike, going to the gym four times a week, swimming, tai chi, yoga, or pool therapy.

Get More Restful Sleep

Sleep is an important time for the brain. The brain will struggle to function properly when neurons become overworked and don't have sufficient opportunity to recuperate. Chapter 5, "Sleep Disruption," discusses in detail the importance of restful sleep as well as techniques to achieve it.

Different levels of brain activity change in each stage of sleep, including REM and non-REM sleep, and certain patterns provide the most restorative sleep. This, in turn, enhances most types of cognitive function. Proper brain activity patterns facilitate mental recovery and unlock cognitive benefits. They foster attention and concentration and enhance learning. They support most aspects of thinking, including memory, problem-solving, creativity, emotional processing, and judgment. Restorative sleep can boost both short- and long-term cognitive performance and help to prevent cognitive decline, no matter what the cause. A regular routine, good sleep hygiene, a dark room, and a habit of building in some winding-down time can all support quality sleep.

Monitor Your Brain Health

It is important to work to maintain optimal brain health as another way to prevent or minimize pain's impact on cognitive functioning. There are a number of ways to approach this, including mental stimulation, physical exercise, a healthy diet, healthy blood pressure, proper blood sugar and cholesterol levels, sunlight exposure for vitamin D, building strong emotional connections to others, meditation, and avoiding smoking and excessive caffeine.

In addition, the human brain can change structurally and functionally with experience and use. This can help or undermine healthy cognitive functioning. Unexplained pain can cause your brain to rewire, sending pain signals where there is no injury and adding to your cognitive problems. To prevent this, you'll need to analyze and address all the collateral damages you've experienced and assess how they have added to your pain. Successfully taking on the challenge of your collateral damages can enhance cognitive functioning.

Avoid Smoking

If you want to avoid a significant contributor to chronic pain, put out that cigarette. Smoking affects the brain, leading to cognitive deficits in auditory, verbal, and visual spatial learning, visual spatial memory, cognitive efficiency, executive skills, general intelligence, and processing speed. It affects the way the brain responds to pain and seems to make people less resilient to an episode of pain. Smokers are three times more likely than nonsmokers to develop chronic back pain. Behavioral interventions, such as smoking cessation programs or medication to ease the effects of withdrawal, can help.

Chapter 9

Chronic Stress

Chronic pain typically creates chronic stress. Why? Because it involves significant, often unending, threats to your needs. When these threats continue unabated, or are minimized or overlooked, they begin to have physical impacts that can undermine your recovery. I have seen many treatment interventions fail when these impacts weren't sufficiently factored into treatment.

Stress negatively impacts both physical and cognitive health. But what is stress? Stress is not an emotion but a state that you enter into when significant needs are at risk. When you are in this state, you will experience a great deal of anxiety and anger. If you don't successfully resolve the threats to your needs, you will remain in that state of stress, which activates the autonomic nervous system, Physical effects of this include increases in heart and respiratory rate, blood pressure, muscle tension, breathing, digestion, and other motor functions. This is known as the fight-or-flight response. Prolonged, chronic stress can cause changes to behavior and damage to your physical and cognitive state and functioning.

ALTERED PERCEPTION

Perception is the cognitive ability to capture, process, and actively make sense of the information that our senses receive. It is a cognitive process that makes it possible to interpret our surroundings and all stimuli and data from the environment. Because pain is regulated by the nervous system, the brain and its cognitive processes are key players in how we perceive pain. If your cognitive functions are undermined by pain, it will alter and distort your perception of events. This alteration in perception can undermine your understanding of your pain, how it's affected you, and what you will need to deal with it. When this happens, it can perpetuate stress. Often my clients will tell me that they are frustrated and feel helpless and hopeless. This distorted way of perceiving their chronic pain situation actually adds to their stress because it suggests that there's no way they can successfully reduce or eliminate the threats to their needs. As you will see in the Recovery section, this perception is not accurate to reality.

DISTORTED FILTERING

The perception of pain is both a sensory and an emotional experience. These experiences are *filtered* through genetics; developmental and social learning experiences; familial, marital, and social status; home and work environments; and cultural variables. These filters vary in status and in how they affect pain perception.

Chronic pain, with its multitude of collateral damages, creates alterations to your filters, as does the use of excessive attention, negative expectations, and negative, distorted appraisals of your situation. Your filters are also influenced by your emotional state. For example, anxiety, anger, depression, and stress will have a negative impact on these filters. Stress hormones and muscle tension are activated in reaction to stress, and higher levels increase your vulnerability to pain.

As you can see, many factors can undermine your ability to filter pain signals. These factors distort what might be the objectively expected pain from your injury.

COMPROMISED IMMUNITY

Stress affects all your physical systems. The body's most basic defenses may even be compromised, as chronic stress can suppress the immune system. Unresolved stress, in fact, can cause the immune system to work *against* the body instead of protecting it. Chronic stress can make you more vulnerable to infections like the common cold and influenza. Chronic stress has been associated with cardiovascular problems, tension headaches, peptic ulcers, hives, asthma, infertility, post-menstrual syndrome, irritable bowel syndrome, and migraines.

RECOVERY: STRESS REDUCTION AND MANAGEMENT

Stress management techniques are numerous. The seven listed below include some typical approaches that are time-tested and very helpful. They also include some approaches that are newer and evolved out of my practice with chronic pain clients. Some of this work is just good general self-care, and some is best done with the help of a trained counselor.

The strategies focus on an in-depth understanding of what stress and chronic pain are all about, and how they are related to the damage to your body and to the state of your needs, your whole life. Some stress management skills were also included in previous Recovery sections, such as looking at life as an athletic event and adjusting to a new normal. Although designed to help minimize physical loss, these skills are also emotionally and psychologically empowering and can add greatly to your ability to cope and manage stress.

Begin by trying to assess what is *most* stressful to you in your pain experience. This will help you identify what targets and techniques will work most effectively.

The strategies described in this section are some common, and common-sense, ways to think about what's stressful and tackle those stressors. Consider it a resource guide. (Some of these techniques will be covered in greater depth in part 3.)

Avail Yourself of Support Groups

Sharing your feelings with people who have had experiences like yours is invaluable. The hunger to feel truly understood in your suffering is a need most people with chronic pain have, and most never satisfy. It is said that the only thing worse than suffering is suffering alone. You need not only to be understood but to have your experience acknowledged and validated. It may be hard to understand why chronic pain affects you as much as it does. You may even doubt your own efforts at recovery. Support groups have the power to help with these issues, just through others sharing their experiences.

I have witnessed the power of such interaction in groups and classes I've run. They offer many benefits. First, support groups can significantly reduce the stress of alienation and negative self-talk that you may experience. Second, they help you feel less alone and can give you new ideas to help cope with your pain. Third, listening to others and being helpful to them is energizing and de-stressing.

Start a Pain Journal

Chronic pain is energy draining and distracting. You may do your best not to think about it, which is understandable. However, this may make it hard for you to talk to others about it. If you can get yourself to keep a journal about your experience, it can help you vent your feelings and reflect on what's happening to you, thereby reducing your stress. Doing this may also give you more information about what you're up against and what helps. Your journal can also help you inform your providers as well as monitor your own progress.

Prioritize What's Meaningful

It's very stressful to wake each day to the same old cycle of pain, limitation, and suffering. To change this, it will be necessary to redesign and restructure your days to make your new day something you can look forward to, instead of being full of fear.

Chronic pain is a thief. It steals your activities and energy. But there are things you can do to restore the balance. Make the effort, no matter how hard, to do things of personal value and importance as often as possible. This will be energizing and de-stressing. As hard as it may seem, try to find reasons to be grateful for being alive. Ask yourself: What's great about my life today? What am I able to do for others? Who and what am I genuinely thankful for in my life?

> "Don't put your energy into your suffering — envision a day that is worth living."

This gets easier if you can see each day as still having value, as an opportunity to find a way to have more of a life. So, inventory what you can do for the day that is meaningful to you — and include that in your Plan A-B-C-D-E (see chapter 6, "Physical De-Activation"). Don't put your energy into your obstacles, your limitations, and your physical suffering. Instead, envision a day that is worth living.

For example, one of my clients decided to engage in random acts of being helpful to others. She looked for opportunities she could respond to; for instance, she helped someone older than her cross the street. She donated to additional charities. She looked for opportunities to pay compliments, and attempted to have positive interactions with everyone she encountered. She found these acts made her feel happy and energized, which reduced her pain and stress.

Think of all the potential positive-energy-creating experiences you may have available to you, despite your pain: Read a book, draw a picture, play a musical instrument, study a new subject online, talk to a friend.

Make Efforts to Stay Connected

Even though you may want to isolate, feeling exiled is a powerful stressor. To counter this, try to be with other people in meaningful ways. Build into your plans time to see friends and family, to interact, even if your time and ability are limited, even if you have to do it online. Seek new relationships. Do volunteer work or any other activity that has positive personal meaning for you, especially if it involves others.

Chronic pain challenges the stability of potentially all your relationships. Your connection to significant others is foundational for your resistance to stress and your power to cope. But you can redesign your relationships to accommodate your new normal and maintain balance and connection. As hard as it may be, work on being a positive role model for your family, friends, or co-workers.

> **"Redesign your relationships to accommodate your new normal and maintain balance and connection."**

Chronic pain can also challenge any sense of empowerment you had before you were injured. It can shake your faith and undermine your values and any positive sense of who you are. This is stress on an existential level. (More will be said about this in chapter 14, "Existential Impacts.") So, in addition to staying connected with others, also stay connected to sources of your personal power. These may be based on faith, philosophy, particular people, or certain activities. Resist a loss of faith in yourself in whatever ways work for you.

Chronic pain may limit your more stimulating activities and make you susceptible to boredom, which, along with being burdened with too many tasks that seem overwhelming or without meaning, can further undermine coping. Lack of stimulation is a core stressor for people. Do what you can to counter this and stay connected — not just to people but also to your interests. Pursue alternate activities that stimulate your soul and accommodate your limits. This may require getting even more flexible and creative, and occasionally doing things outside your comfort zone.

Cultivate New Ways of Communicating

Not being able to communicate your needs can be a big stressor. My clients often say, "I don't know how to talk about what I want or need; I don't know how to communicate my experience." You may find this to be true for you too. Perhaps your efforts leave you feeling scattered, confused, or self-critical. Perhaps you think you don't deserve help, or you think, "I'm a failure and it's all my fault."

You may need to change how you think about your pain and how you talk to yourself. You may need to reinvent your methods of communicating with yourself and others. Many of my clients are uncomfortable with expressing vulnerability, anxiety, anger, and depression; they fear being a burden if they are too candid about what they want or need. However, the willingness to try can be extremely important to managing your stress.

Communication with others is enhanced by the quality of your interaction with yourself. The key here is to be open and vulnerable with yourself about the reality of your experience, how much you've been harmed, and how much you are suffering. Be accepting of your needs and seek to communicate them unequivocally to others who can help. Be compassionate with yourself, and liberate yourself to share your experience without shame, guilt, or anxiety.

> "Relaxation, fun, and leisure are no less important than work. Make them a bigger part of your daily routine."

You may think others don't have the experience to appreciate what you're going through or to understand it, but everyone has experienced physical pain and emotional suffering of some kind. Most people have had some version of these experiences that is prolonged or even chronic. Help the people around you understand by making reference to their own experience.

Make Time

Stress is better managed for everyone if you seek balance in what you need and want to do. Schedules with too little downtime always create more stress. This is even more likely when living with chronic pain, because of its impact on getting things done. Take the time to examine your daily routine and modify it for balance. Nose to the grindstone with little regard for your level of stress makes it worse, so identify what you need to find balance. Perhaps it is better organization and time management. The most effective way to manage time is to find ways to get more done in less time. Be creative and innovative! Sometimes it is learning to say no, and to be more realistic in your expectations. Relaxation, fun, and leisure are no less important than work. Make them a bigger part of your daily routine.

Use Time-Honored Approaches

Seek professional evaluation and counseling in stress management from a mental health professional — a therapist also with expertise in pain management. This, along with following your physician's advice, is the most common approach to stress management. Stress in chronic pain is often extreme, and when it is, your emotional and psychological suffering requires at least as much attention as your physical suffering, to mitigate the frustration, anger, resentment, anxiety, and depression that can go hand in hand with your stress.

Here are some more of the most reliable ways to manage stress:

Hypnotherapy is a long-established approach to pain and stress management. Hypnosis can implant suggestions, such as, "You're going to sleep soundly tonight, and you'll have less pain." This approach can be learned and practiced at home.

Exercise, regularly planned, measured, and slightly physically challenging, can significantly help to better manage stress. Under the guidance of a physical therapist or trainer versed in chronic pain, you can integrate into your life a program of activity suitable to your abilities.

Diet and nutritional balance can help reduce stress. Eat regular and healthy meals. As best you can, eat natural foods (lots of fruits, vegetables, whole grains, etc.).

Caffeine-free living can also help. The stimulants in coffee, black teas, cola drinks, chocolate, some over-the-counter pain medications, and other foods and drugs can intensify your anxiety, stress, and pain. Consuming too much caffeine is like trying to put a fire out by throwing gasoline on it.

Mind-body techniques are plentiful; explore and see which approach best suits you. Techniques such as yoga, tai chi, qigong, guided imagery, and meditation can all help you to relax and decrease stress levels in significant ways. Once you have learned these techniques, you can do them on your own at any time throughout your day.

Quiet breathing is a simple, free, and accessible form of self-care. For the simplest form, sit or lie quietly and observe your breathing without trying to control it. If pain or thoughts are distracting, simply notice them without pushing them away. Think of them as clouds passing over; then return to observing your breath. Do this for about twenty minutes. You can also add imagery. Breathe calmly while you imagine a tranquil scene in which you feel comfortable, safe, and relaxed. Include colors, sounds, smells, and your feelings. Do this for five to ten minutes each day. Another technique is four-square breathing: Inhale to a count of four, hold for a count of four, exhale to a count of four, then hold to a count of four. Inhale and exhale fully so that your abdomen expands and contracts like a balloon with each breath. Repeat for up to ten cycles. (Stop if you feel light-headed: Don't go beyond your own physical and emotional comfort level.)

There is a world of support out there for reducing stress, and many free or affordable resources online, in YouTube videos, newsletters, social media groups, and email lists, for a home-based stress-management plan. Look for something that works for you and let yourself see it as a "get to" rather than a "have to" — a resource rather than one more burden. Simple new habits can have powerful effects.

Chapter 10

Psychological Challenges

Everything I have shared in this book so far has been part of a process of discovery with my clients. A process of trying to understand what it is (in addition to an initial injury) that contributes to the pain they have, what kind of suffering it produces and how much, and how they might maximize the success of treatment. The physical impacts from injury and pain are easier to understand than the emotional and psychological impacts. But it's important to remind yourself that anything that negatively affects your personhood has to be considered in your quest to understand and master your pain. This chapter focuses on how you may feel, emotionally and psychologically, about the way you've been physically impacted by your pain.

As you read this chapter, consider your feelings and thoughts in context of the physical impacts discussed in the previous chapters. Think about what needs may be threatened, and what added stress and disempowerment your physical impacts may produce.

The physical impacts of chronic pain lead to physical limitations and additional damages to the body, which in turn can damage your sense of physical identity, self-image, self-worth, and self-confidence. This can add to pain, suffering, and the feeling of being overwhelmed and helpless. It makes it harder to access your innate potential to help yourself.

Facing a threat to your sense of self — your self-image and physical identity, your feelings of self-worth, and your level of confidence in the world — is the existential equivalent of facing a bear in the woods. Together they can produce extreme, potentially overwhelming anxiety. So you see why it's important to prevent or address such threats. Fortunately, even here there are recovery tools that can minimize or even eliminate the impacts.

DAMAGED PHYSICAL IDENTITY

One of the pillars of self is physical identity. If this identity changes in a negative sense, for example with disfigurement, age, or injury, there may be a negative impact on your sense of self. This can in turn have a big impact on your experience of social acceptance and inclusion — and your perceptions of how others view you.

In general, physical intactness, competence, and attractiveness derive importance from their relationship to survival. Societal attitudes tend to reinforce a positive sense of identity and esteem in individuals with physical attractiveness, health, strength, or athletic prowess. Given this, many people find it hard to hold onto their personal worth and identity as something distinct from their physical ability or condition. This is likely even more true for those who identify with being physically fit or an athlete.

Psychological tests, used in conjunction with measures of physical damage and loss of function, reveal that the impact on identity can be extreme.

Signs and symptoms of identity loss include:

- Negative self-talk
- Lack of confidence
- Uncontrollable negative thoughts
- Self-doubt

An athlete, whose identity is often closely tied in with their physical strength and skill, often perceives chronic injury as a life-or-death matter. If you tend to have a higher athletic identity, you're more apt to experience depressive reactions after injury than someone with less of an athletic identity. The more you identify with athletic performance or general physical strength and competence, the less stable your individual identity and self-esteem may become as you face an injury or chronic pain. This may lead to you seeing yourself in a new and negative way — as "damaged goods."

RUPTURED SELF-IMAGE

Part of our identity is based on self-image. A fundamental form of suffering in chronic pain is the loss of self-image, sometimes perceived as crumbling away due to the physical impact of your pain. What you need is the simultaneous development of an equally valued self-image that is *not* dependent upon your physical state. Without that, the sense of loss and psychological impact can be devastating.

This loss of self can start early — sometimes even before a diagnosis is made — and it continues to grow insidiously from there.

When you're forced to limit normal activities to protect your health and deteriorating physical state, you do so at great cost to your self-image. Living a restricted life can foster an all-consuming retreat into an image of yourself as a *patient*, and somehow no longer a *person*.

John, a client of mine with severe chronic back pain, who was continuing to deteriorate physically at the time, once commented, "My broken body cost me my membership in society. It made me drop out of life, and left me feeling like an outcast."

Like John, you may be reduced to living marginally, leaving your prior social worlds entirely, and losing your sense of belonging in them. Chronic pain's impacts can flood identity. It and your physical limitations can become the focus of your life, and if you judge yourself by yardsticks more appropriately applied to the healthy and able, you may no longer feel a member of that society. The world seems structured for them, a club you can no longer participate in. Your self-image now revolves around dysfunction and disability.

ERODED SELF-WORTH

Chronic pain has a way of entering your life and draining you of feelings of worthiness. Pain and physical limitations obstruct your efforts to meet life goals, and this can have a disastrous effect on self-worth. The physical impacts from chronic pain alone make outcomes like these more likely:

- Inability to complete educational programs and meet educational goals
- Loss of jobs and career opportunities
- Unstable or failed relationships
- Estrangement from or poor/unsupportive relationships with friends and family members

- Inability to be financially self-supporting
- Inability to take part in community activities
- Cognitive and emotional difficulties

When you perceive yourself as being unable to do anything worthwhile, you may label yourself as "worthless." This further erodes your self-esteem. Feeling worthless for long periods of time may lead to clinical depression.

Anyone in your life who reinforces your sense of diminished worth due to your physical limitations is not helping. It's up to you to challenge the notion that the circumstances of your physical state should determine your worth.

Sally, a client of mine and a senior corporate officer, captured the issue when she said, "I used to feel like I could do anything. It was easy for me to build myself up if I had a presentation or walked into a roomful of strangers. But now, I feel like I'm not as 'worthy' as I once was. I look different, I can't do the things I once did, and worst of all, I feel different. I'm not the same person I was before my injury."

Now, when you park in the disabled spot—despite the glares—or use a cane that draws glances or stares, it can feel as if someone has delivered a blow to your self-esteem. Body image and physical limitations can cause great confusion with self-esteem. In our society we put much emphasis on our outward appearance. But the effects of lack of exercise and activity, combined with the side effects of medications, may give you a body that you are neither comfortable in nor proud of. This can make you feel diminished, marginalized, and even discriminated against.

In many parts of American culture, if chronic pain has brought with it a weight gain, this can exacerbate a negative self-image. As my client Anne observed, "Oh, how I miss that old me who once enjoyed shopping for clothes. Now it even hurts to get dressed." Pain, she explained, caused her to quickly exchange beauty for comfort when it came to clothing. But along with that, she said, "I exchanged my pride with a lower self-image. I'm just so eager to make another exchange! It's like hell to live with a body that you don't feel pride in, a body which causes daily frustrations."

Social isolation also contributes to negative self-esteem, as Tina commented:

> *"After I was diagnosed with chronic fatigue syndrome, I let everything go. I stopped exercising, I quit my clubs. I lost friends because I kept canceling plans. I quit volunteering. I also lost my sense of worth, though, because I wasn't receiving praise from anyone any longer."*

Ultimately, as your sense of self-worth erodes, the following disempowering behaviors often arise:

- Heavy self-criticism and overall dissatisfaction
- Hypersensitivity to criticism and feelings of being attacked, along with resentment against the perceived critics
- Chronic indecision and an exaggerated fear of mistakes
- Excessive will to please and unwillingness to displease anyone
- Overcompensation, trying to hard to find ways to feel good about yourself, which can lead to frustration when it doesn't achieve the desired outcomes
- Guilt and dwelling on or exaggerating the magnitude of things that don't go well with others
- Floating hostility and general defensiveness and irritability (with or without provocation)
- Pessimism and a general negative outlook
- Envy or general resentment of others who don't have your problems
- Perceiving temporary setbacks as permanent, intolerable conditions

DIMINISHED SELF-CONFIDENCE

People with self-confidence generally agree that the following statements are true:

- I can always manage to solve difficult problems if I try hard enough.
- If someone opposes me, I can find means and ways to get what I want.
- It's easy for me to stick to my aims and accomplish my goals.
- I feel that I can deal efficiently with unexpected events.
- I know how to handle unforeseen situations.
- I can solve most problems if I invest the necessary effort.
- I can remain calm in family difficulties because I can rely on my coping abilities.
- When I am confronted with a problem, I can usually find several solutions.
- No matter what comes my way, I am usually able to handle it.

Chronic pain, with its multiple physical impacts, can radically alter these statements in a negative direction. This erodes self-confidence. And without self-confidence, responding to changes in your life becomes harder.

It becomes more taxing to find motivation and make effort. It becomes tougher to increase your level of effort toward change or to decide to change your goals. You may increasingly avoid difficult tasks. You may feel defeated by challenge, and experience it as revealing your shortcomings. You'll become reluctant to face failures or setbacks and more inclined to give up. You'll be less likely to set challenging goals for yourself and less committed to each goal. You'll be less likely to be persistent, goal-setting, and high-performing.

With low self-confidence, in sharp contrast to your pre-injury state, you may fall into a depressed state and respond to any changes in your environment with a lack of belief in your own abilities. Ultimately, your physical limitations may leave you feeling helpless: that all efforts are pointless, that all tasks are impossible.

RECOVERY: DEEPENING YOUR SENSE OF SELF

You have the power to deal with the physical impact of chronic pain on how you see yourself — if you are willing to reconsider how you define your losses. *You get to choose* whether or not you have really lost your identity in the context of your new physical reality.

This often requires a level of contemplation and self-exploration that many people have never even considered. If you are willing to do this, start by asking yourself: *What are the key attributes of who I am?* Understand: It is possible to view physical performance as something you do, rather than who you are.

Identity based on physical prowess is, by its very nature, unstable and prone to variability. An injury that disrupts physical performance is only one of an inevitable number of physical changes that all of us will most likely experience in our lifetimes as we age.

Let's put the challenge to your sense of physical identity in proper perspective. Consider your values, your goals, and your philosophy as to what it is that makes people matter. If you and your significant other, family, and friends value and identify your physical condition as who you *are*, then the damage caused by physical losses may be unavoidable and psychologically traumatic. However, if you think about all that makes up who you are, you will likely see that no one feature defines you as a person. What you cannot *do* is surely a loss. But who you *are* cannot be lost, unless you yourself forget all you know about what makes you who you are.

If you can tap into a greater awareness of yourself instead of focusing on the smaller trauma, you will experience an accompanying sense of challenge. You will seek to maintain and preserve yourself by accessing all that you are despite your limitations. Your identity is defined by you, your greater self, not by circumstance.

There are multiple ways to express who you are. There are multiple ways to be physically competent. Physical capacity, as part of identity, must be placed in context to be appreciated. This next story epitomizes that.

Years ago, Mr. Soto, a fifty-year-old martial arts instructor, was hit by a car that was going eighty miles per hour. His body was so broken that he was in a near full-body cast.

Mr. Soto had been practicing karate since he was a child. Before the accident, his routine was to train hard every day for many hours. Several days after the accident, a friend visited him at the hospital. Mr. Soto informed his friend that he must get back to the dojo, to teach his students and to train. His friend said, "You'll be lucky to get out of this bed, let alone be able to train!" Mr. Soto replied, "I am training now," and showed the several fingers of his right hand, outside the cast, that he was repeatedly flexing. Mr. Soto indicated that this was his practice now, and it would extend to whatever parts of him became available to him as he healed.

Two years later, Mr. Soto, despite all the odds against him, was back teaching and training at his dojo. Mr. Soto's recovery was based on his understanding that because of the accident, those finger movements, and all that followed, were the equivalent effort to the training he used to do. *He* was not diminished; his identity was not lost. He was still an individual who trained hard.

Finding this deeper sense of self and identity is part of your individual spirituality and values. Your successes and failures and how you do things do not define you. Try to keep performance in context and keep performance distinct from your identity. This allows you to retain your sense of who you are.

Here are four strategies toward recovery of your sense of self.

Reclaim Your Physical Being

Do you need to be fully functional physically to earn a good sense of self? Do you have to be able to do certain things in a certain way? Work to shift from a doing identity to a being identity. To do this, *express who you are physically in whatever way you can*. Create a new physical self in alignment with your limitations but also in keeping with your values — like overcoming limits, exceeding expectations, and operating at the same level of self-challenge.

You can you feel good about yourself, regardless of your limitations, by understanding what you really are: infinite potential. And by appreciating that your *intentions* — not your achievements — and how committed you are to them, are at the heart of self-satisfaction.

This is the dichotomy of *being*, where self-worth is internally determined, versus *doing*, where self-worth is determined by an external source. Athletic performance is an example of an external source on which someone might depend for a positive sense of self. On the other hand, an athlete who acknowledges their value regardless of performance level is basing a positive sense of self on an individual, internal value — distinct from, and not dependent on, athletic performance.

Redefine Your Self-Worth

Personal worth is innate: We can feel our worth by understanding it is based on what we are as human beings, not who we are at any moment.

> "Know that there is always a way to feel good about yourself, no matter what happens to you."

What we are is infinite potential driven by evolutionary forces. This was discussed at length in the introduction, "From Mystery to Mastery." But for most of us, we feel like our sense of worth needs to be earned, that it's dependent on whether or not the person we think we are is adequate to qualify us for self-worth. There is a difference between appreciating yourself and having a sense of worth.

So, it's not the attributes we acquire, or our values around them, that should determine how we feel about ourselves. Our attributes and values may be about achievement or about character, status, success, or other valued human goals. Remember, you have choice about who you are. *We can always change who we are. What we are only requires expression.* It is the true driving force for what we value most about each other.

When a good sense of self is contingent on a specific performance or achievement, it is unstable. While you should value the qualities that define who you truly are, beyond performance, when your value is based on *what* you are, it is permanent. Chronic pain may challenge who you are, but it cannot take "you" away unless you are willing to give up on yourself. When you are struggling with that challenge, there will be a tendency toward negative self-talk and reduced self-value, a source of great existential stress.

Knowing yourself as well as you can will help you better understand what you find most motivating in life. What matters to you is most important. This includes being aware of your behaviors and performance, but not inexorably linking your self-esteem to your difficulty in expressing what motivates you. Your personal value is distinct from performance, accomplishments, or behavior. Not being able to perform does not diminish your worth.

Know that there is always a way to feel good about yourself, no matter what happens to you. It is in how you meet the challenges chronic pain throws at you that you reveal your sense of self-worth. Feeling good about yourself begins with understanding that, as a product of evolution, you have inherent potential to deal with any challenges in your life. To adapt, to survive, and even to thrive. It means appreciating what matters to you and your drive to express it. Understanding that self-worth is not determined by anything about your life that is transient.

Feeling good about yourself revolves around the understanding that you have the power to choose, to shape, and to form your life into supporting what's most important to you. The tools of self-discovery and of your existential immune system discussed throughout this book will enable you to accomplish this.

Restore Your Self-Image

Your perception of yourself depends on how you choose to view changes in your physical state or life circumstances. Who you are remains intact — but you may lose touch with that reality if you get angry and anxious about what has changed in your life. If you can maintain perspective, you'll refrain from condemning yourself for any loss of performance or appearance. Then you may see the truth and power you have to contend with what has changed.

Your self-image is based on your intrinsic value, not some set of physical circumstances you find yourself in. Over the course of a lifetime, who will you be when you are no longer fully physically competent? There is so much more to you as a person.

Positive self-image leads to positive self-talk, creativity, and inspiration. While injury negatively affects performance, it is also an opportunity to affirm your self-image by challenging yourself to evolve, to transform, to manifest who you are, and what your goals are, in the myriad ways this can be accomplished.

People who care about you can be instrumental in validating your self-acceptance and self-esteem. Is your love for someone based on what they can and cannot do? Would you value the opinion of anyone who thinks less of you due to your physical limitations? It's important that everyone focus on treating you first as a valued individual, not a diagnosis.

It is often difficult when people don't understand your pain and suffering. No matter your injury, the true extent of harm done to you may seem invisible, which makes it harder for your family and friends to perceive it.

> "We must, in a very positive way, determine who we are and trust our definitions."

They may not believe that you are in pain; they might dump guilt on top of your pain. This can lead to deeper feelings of unworthiness. However, this book offers many ways to undo or prevent this from happening. This need not be an inevitable outcome.

If people you associate with, including family members, friends, and colleagues, treat you badly, try to correct the situation by explaining the devastating consequences their comments and actions have on you. They may not realize the damage they are causing, and subsequently be able to change their behavior.

So often we tend to give other people the power to determine how we feel about ourselves. We must *not* give away our personal power to anyone. We must *not* let anyone else define who we are. We must, in a very positive way, determine who we are and trust our definitions. The antidote to a negative self-image is to have a strong sense of individual worth that isn't dependent on others' opinions.

To optimize the quality of your life, surround yourself with people who will affirm and validate you in an authentic way. They don't have to agree with everything you do, but they must respect your right to feel good about yourself without condition.

Affirm Your Self-Confidence

You may or may not have been a confident person before chronic pain struck. Nonetheless, pain can undermine what self-confidence you have. To some extent, this is understandable. Much of what you could once do physically may no longer be available to you. But there are many ways to restore your physical confidence, by demonstrating that you can still do things and get things done, albeit in different ways.

There are thousands of examples of people who have done this. Soldiers who have lost limbs; adventurers whose accidents have left them mostly paralyzed; people who have adjusted to an onset of sight or hearing impairment.

Confidence needs to be based on intention, not outcomes. You can be confident that you will *try*. You will give it your best shot and try to figure out how to get it done. You may try multiple ways. You're more likely to envision a positive, confident future as you figure out ways to counter and overcome your limitations. This is highly likely if you are willing to adapt and make modifications.

Tools and Takeaways for Part 3

Approaching life with creativity rather than fear will help you keep your edge and recollect who and what you really are.

The self-assessments in appendix B can help you identify and describe possible personal, existential impacts of chronic pain:

- Personal Experience Inventory
- Personal Impacts Checklist
- Risk Factors for Injury Inventory
- Social-Emotional Impacts Checklist

Bottom Line

How you think and feel about yourself and about your situation, and what meaning you attribute to those thoughts and feelings, affects your pain and fuels your recovery. There is always potential for greater personal strength to arise to meet and neutralize or defeat your suffering.

PART 3

The Personal
Experience

Chapter 11

Day-to-Day Impacts

T his chapter begins our deeper exploration of the damages that can happen to you as a person, beyond what has been covered in earlier chapters. The subsections are organized to give you a holistic, three-dimensional picture of the extent to which these damages can affect different aspects of your life. These damages include impacts that chronic pain has on your day-to-day life, your life situation, your overall functioning, and your ongoing experience — I refer to all of these as *existential pain*. Existential pain is personal: It is all of what happens within you and to you as a person, including your ability to operate cognitively, psychologically, and emotionally. The resulting damages are negative impacts on the totality of what matters to you and what makes you who you are.

You might think this would be obvious to everyone. Unfortunately, it's not. The personal impact of pain, as you can see by the six chapters it will take us to cover it, is complicated and multifaceted. Even in cases when these impacts are considered in a treatment setting, there is often insufficient depth and scope for exploring and accounting for them.

However, while the options for reducing your physical pain through medical interventions may be limited, the options for reducing physical pain by addressing existential suffering are many, and they can be highly effective in reducing not only your pain but your suffering as well.

While you are reading this chapter, you may initially feel overwhelmed by the scope and multiplicity of the potential existential impacts. It can be quite frightening to examine the true depth and extent of your losses.

And it would be understandable if at first you experience this information as an additional burden. But if you are willing to explore, you will find solutions to all these impacts — solutions that can empower you in ways that might never have happened otherwise. I would never wish the suffering of chronic pain on anyone. But I know that within suffering there is potential for a greater personal strength to arise, as so many of my clients have shown me. I have been exploring the personal impacts of chronic

> **"Meaning is at the true heart of any impact."**

pain from an existential perspective for many years. This means that I do not focus so much on what happened to my clients but rather on what these events mean to them. Meaning is at the true heart of any impact.

Following my discoveries, I prepared a client intake packet that tops sixty-five pages. The packet has evolved to assess a person's most important needs and whether they have been damaged. The most important of these needs are the ones that are not only damaged but that matter a great deal to you and to who you are. Understanding the subtleties of these personal impacts can explain much about chronic pain and reveal powerful potential areas for enhancing recovery.

However, these impacts are not easy to measure. The intake packet is designed to reveal them through a pattern analysis — a careful look at all the items measured to reach an in-depth understanding of who you are in a multidimensional way. One thing I know is that the elements of your existential needs are far more extensive than many people consider. I have learned this from my clients over the past twenty years, as we explored together the meaning pain has taken on in their life. The list of impacts keeps growing — and so do the options for recovery.

THE MESSAGE IN MEANING

To begin to understand personal impacts of any kind, consider that we all experience what happens to us in a unique way, against the backdrop of who we are and what we need. The situations chronic pain creates do not spell out what impacts we will experience and to what extent they will matter. So, how do you go about exploring meaning and individual differences? This is best accomplished by first examining the foundational information:

- Who you are
- Where you were in your life when you were injured
- Your life history
- The extent of your losses

This careful examination will help you define and understand how you are experiencing what has happened to you. Whether you understand your pain to be minimal, impactful, or at a crisis level, this examination of meaning will reveal if it has created significant threats to your essential needs.

> "This is 'slow trauma,' and it is something you can only understand by looking across time at the patterns of your experience."

A meaning-based analysis considers the context — *your* context — for the pain experience. Pain scales that ask you to rate your pain on a 0 to 10 scale rarely take into consideration whether you are an athlete, a stay-at-home parent, a police officer, or an individual with little previous experience dealing with pain. Yet these different backgrounds can powerfully affect the meaning that you attribute to your pain, how you experience it, and how much you are bothered and disrupted by it! For example, police officers, firefighters, and soldiers are trained to think about pain differently. They may experience an injury as troublesome, but they are motivated to complete the mission despite the pain. To keep on fighting. You and I, in the same situation, might experience the same injury as calamitous and disabling. We are each unique, and individual differences matter.

It's important to recognize that the life impacts described in this chapter can change your perception of your entire life. You will need to come to understand how they combine and how they reshape you — often in ways that multiply the individual impacts.

Depending on the meaning you attribute to the existential impacts of pain, they can be minimal or they can suck the life out of you, if your coping system isn't up to the task of managing them. And meaningful existential threats make it harder for you to access your innate abilities to combat them. Like an uncontrolled forest fire, these threats can multiply the losses you suffer. This is the "slow trauma" I mentioned in chapter 3, "Injury and Collateral Damages," and it is something you can only understand by looking across time at the patterns of your experience. When you don't recognize or attend to this, anxiety, anger, depression, chronic stress, and grief may follow. But when you acknowledge and embrace the importance of these threats, you hold the possibility of gaining energy and personal power to fight back and reclaim your life.

There is much in our day-to-day personal experience we may only become aware of, or feel the importance of, when it goes away. So, as you review each potential personal impact in this chapter and the chapters that follow, take your time. Identify what may apply to you. You will find in the Recovery sections specific information about how to address, counter, or correct each of these personal impacts of chronic pain.

LOSS OF THE ORDINARY

In my practice I see people from many walks of life: carpenters and lawyers, doctors and technology experts, athletes and ballet dancers, business-people and brokers, homemakers and captains of industry. Like most of us, they take their day-to-day lives for granted. Human beings prefer a sense of fundamental predictability to what we do, and to the patterns of how things happen in our lives. Anyone who has been through a life-altering experience can tell you how traumatic it can be to have that sense of the ordinary torn away.

Chronic pain is different; though not a sudden experience, over time it is no less life-altering than an earthquake or a tornado. This confuses people. With chronic pain, experienced by most as a creeping sense of dread rather than an obvious obliteration of all that is familiar, people often don't realize that their basic sense of place and security in the world is threatened until it's gone. Chronic pain eats away at it like slow-acting acid. It produces enormous alterations in the landscapes of ordinary life, tangible and intangible.

How do most people react to this?

At first you try to continue to live your life as normally as possible. As pain permeates all the nooks and crannies of your life, however, it begins to interfere with your usual routines and activities. You begin to question your ability to follow everyday routines. Self-care, chores, tasks, work, exercise, creativity, entertainment, socializing, and recreation—all become challenging, often undoable. Making plans or managing expectations becomes difficult or impossible. Dealing with your pain becomes more important than getting things done. Your life begins to look like a heap of good intentions, constantly undone by your latest pain flare-up. Your sense of "life as usual" and "everything is okay" evaporates, replaced by a mounting sense of loss and powerful negative emotions: anxiety, anger, and sadness, which often end in deep depression.

People need continuity in their lives. Continuity in your life includes the things that happen on a regular basis and are predictable. When the only ordinary, predictable thing in your life is the likelihood of ongoing pain and failed activities, you may increasingly feel like one of my clients: "When the pain didn't go away, I felt lost and adrift."

UNPREDICTABILITY

Chronic pain also makes life unpredictable. Moment to moment, you're not sure how you'll feel or what you'll be able to do. You don't know if you'll be able to tolerate or control your pain. You are constantly forced to contend with unfamiliar limitations, modify your behavior, abandon tasks and activities, and change plans, and you can never be certain how things will work out.

When this happens, you may feel as if everything that matters is slipping from your grasp. You think you're losing control of your life. Your ability to work, and to attend to the day-to-day business of your life, becomes increasingly less certain. The only predictable thing becomes the likelihood of a life that feels less valuable, productive, and satisfying.

> "Uncertainty toward most things in your life is itself an existential threat, and profoundly stressful."

Sometimes, when you look in the mirror, you see someone you're not sure you recognize. You may frequently change your lifestyle to adapt to your ever-burgeoning pain condition. You may have to let go of hopes and dreams. You are left mourning the loss of the person you once were. What might you lose next?

Uncertainty toward most things in your life is itself an existential threat, and profoundly stressful.

This doesn't just apply to what you can do physically. Your ability to participate meaningfully in your current relationships becomes uncertain as well. Part of this is caused by the changes in your emotional and physical state that affect how you react to others, and how they react to you. People you care about may face unwanted adjustments and losses to their lives. This is how chronic pain can cause major conflicts and relationship stress. If these issues are not resolved, you may lose once-supportive relationships. Ultimately, these changes may leave you uncertain about the future of all your relationships.

UNDERMINED SENSE OF WELL-BEING AND SAFETY

With chronic pain, nothing in your life — in your physical or emotional states — feels balanced or safe. Ordinary activity and movement become minefields for potential harm. Pain begins to be perceived as uncontrolled danger. The roles, activities, and relationships that provided you with a sense of well-being, safety, stability, and grounding begin to erode as the stress of your condition heightens. As you become flooded by anxiety and anger from threats to numerous needs, your ability to cope declines. This can cause you to lose confidence that you can keep yourself safe in any meaningful way or feel a sense of security or well-being.

VIOLATED VALUES

People often don't think about how pain impacts us in light of the typical values held in our society: ambition, capability, hard work, competence, effectiveness, courage, achievement, integrity, honesty, imagination, intelligence, independence, self-reliance, self-sufficiency, responsibility, dependability, reliability, rationality, self-control, self-discipline, helpfulness, open-mindedness, and being forgiving and loving. How likely is it that your pain could violate your relationship to any or all of these: ambition, capability, competence, effectiveness, independence, self-reliance, and self-sufficiency?

People also don't necessarily consider how important their values are until those values are challenged. Yet values are important to your sense of success in living. They represent what you believe in and aspire to be. Therefore, a violation of your values is a violation of you as a person.

CHALLENGE TO MEANING

Our internal self, or subjective life, is where our sense of meaning and purpose live. Chronic pain can redefine that inner self—to that of a patient, a sufferer, a person with an undermined sense of selfhood and significance. The functional impacts of your pain can damage your ability to feel a sense of purpose or value, or to think you can have an impact in your world.

When everything that once defined you in your relationship with the rest of the world is threatened, it becomes much harder to feel good about yourself. Chronic pain has the power to make you feel meaningless, both in the present and in contemplation of a future filled with continuing and compounding loss.

ALIENATION FROM OTHERS

People with chronic pain often come to my practice feeling alone in their suffering, alienated, and ashamed. Like them, you may have been made to feel like an object, a number, an experiment, or worse still, a faker and a fraud. You may think your physical and emotional pain is not understood by your providers, significant others, family, and friends. You may even be biased against yourself by thinking, "I should have been more successful at recovering."

Have you been reluctant to share your physical or emotional discomfort with others? You may believe it would be a burden to them if they knew how much you hurt, so you don't complain. You may believe that if you share your suffering, they will reject you. You may expect to be met with skepticism, disbelief, or anger. Unfortunately, this often leads to a situation where, at a time when you need love, compassion, sympathy, and support, you are afraid to seek it, or you see it as weakness.

> "Recovery from feeling alienated begins with an understanding that it is possible for others to get close to understanding your experience."

The truth is, it can be very difficult both for you *and* for the people in your life who *don't* suffer from chronic pain to understand what you are going through. Perhaps until now you've lacked a way to understand chronic pain at the level explored in this book. You may have felt uncomfortable with being vulnerable and open to your needs and the needs of others in your situation. Recovery from feeling alienated begins with an understanding that it is possible for others to get close to understanding your experience.

Don't assume people want to reject or dismiss your suffering. Like you, they may also feel powerless to understand or help.

That can change if you help them help you. What happens when you share your own experience, tell your story? If you do not invite a dialogue with someone else where you give them the chance to care, you miss the chance to discover this. You may be the one who, without knowing it, has marginalized yourself, and even invited others to do the same. In that case, you have shut both yourself and others out. This leaves you believing that you and your pain are invisible to the world, that you do not matter. Or worse still, that maybe you are making too much of it, that maybe you *are* a weakling or a fraud.

When it seems difficult, if not impossible, to receive validation and support from the people you expect to receive it from, including yourself, you find you're suffering so much more. Suffering is hard; suffering alone is so much worse.

BIAS AND DISCRIMINATION FROM FRIENDS

It is not your imagination: People with chronic pain are discriminated against. Some friends, associates, and family, even with the best of intentions, will behave toward you as if you lack the intelligence, skill, or thoughtfulness to manage your own pain. They may presume to

143

understand your condition better than you or your doctors; everybody thinks they're an expert. They may ask questions and make suggestions as if you've been sitting on your hands, doing nothing, letting pain devastate your life. As you struggle to come to terms with your condition and to find a way to recovery, it's often shocking to find others against you. In this way, others' perceptions of your condition, while usually not intended to be hurtful, may make it worse.

This is a powerful form of bias and discrimination that you may suffer, one based on the ignorance of others. They often don't understand how desperate you are to be rid of your pain, the lengths you've gone to in order to deal with it, or the obstacles you've encountered. They do not understand how complicated many chronic pain conditions are. They do not know how common-sense and intelligent approaches to managing your pain will frequently fail due to flaws in the system of care or an underestimation of the impacts of your pain. They may see you as lazy, negligent, hysterical, weak, self-indulgent, or attempting to manipulate your condition for your own gain.

These are biased and misinformed reactions. These views contribute to the loss of social support, the loss of friendships and social life and possibly marriage, and even the loss of job and career. These skewed views may cause you to doubt your own perceptions and efforts. Then you feel guilty or ashamed, or resentful and angry — even cynical — over the apparent lack of empathy and compassion of others.

BIAS AND DISCRIMINATION FROM PROVIDERS

With so many challenges, you've likely turned to medical treatment to save you. We all count on our health care providers to be the ones who get it, the ones who will care for us. We look to them for compassion, effort, and relief. Unfortunately, those things are not always to be found. For those with chronic, medically vexing conditions, attention and sympathy from providers may be absent — even at the outset. But even the providers who are attentive in the beginning are likely to withdraw if you fail to respond to one medical intervention after another.

Often, health care providers feel frustrated and helpless; they don't know how to deal with their inability to help you feel better. People with incurable, irreversible, and progressive conditions, such as degenerative disk and joint disease, may end up having a difficult time even finding health care providers who will take them on as patients.

Consequently, many people with chronic pain find themselves literally "fired" by their treating physicians after a year or so, especially after numerous painful and invasive treatments have been tried and failed. They are left on their own to try and find another doctor.

Is this the fault of the provider? No. Providers who don't understand the complexity of chronic pain as described in this book will be frustrated in their efforts to help you. They won't understand how their medical diagnosis and treatment is part of a larger constellation of contributors to chronic pain, much of which their medical care cannot touch.

When I work with clients, I do my best to understand their medical challenges and the limits of their treatment. I understand that many things are contributing to their pain that are not a result of their structural issues. Because of this, I don't experience the same sense of mystery or frustration that medical providers often do. I can put the value of my efforts into proper context because I understand some of the built-in limitations of physical treatment.

The same cannot be said of medical providers who don't understand the existential model of pain. These providers can end up with a negative attitude or orientation — not because they're judging their patients, but because they really don't understand what they're dealing with and think somehow it must be the fault of the patient. The providers I end up working with are relieved to see the big picture, understand the limits of what they can do for their patients, and appreciate how much more can be done by applying the concepts presented in this book.

Doctors and insurance companies may also use the concept known as *secondary gain* to explain your pain. Secondary gain is the notion that chronic pain is psychological and persists only because the person enjoys one or more "rewards" from suffering. These so-called rewards are considered to be emotional, such as sympathy or monetary support, are said to reinforce the pain, and are often suspected of being or becoming the reason behind partial or complete disability. This is also a biased and misinformed view.

When medical or insurance professionals designate someone's continuing difficulty as a bid for secondary gain, they turn the truth, the reality of the disabled person's existence, upside-down. I would like a ten-dollar bill for every time one of my clients' providers incorrectly accused them of treatment noncompliance or exaggeration. Though this is not an intentional slight, it has the potential to blame the victim and justify the actions of insurance companies, opposing attorneys, and many of the private, county, state, and federal bureaucracies purporting to assist persons with disabilities. The idea, built on stereotypes, of secondary gain can contribute to ongoing discrimination against people disabled by chronic pain.

In my experience with several thousand clients, secondary gain is rarely, if ever, helpful as a concept. Originating with Freud decades ago, the concept has never been rigorously examined. *Secondary loss*, on the other hand, is provable: Your pain can cause tremendous loss in your life, which in turn can trash your efforts to recover.

If you or your providers have used secondary gain to explain your chronic pain, you can harness that as a challenge to everyone to better understand what actually motivates you. Equipped with a deeper understanding of your pain and ways to reduce it, you may be better able to find a provider who will work with you to address your pain.

RECOVERY: REESTABLISHING THE ORDINARY

Our lives change on a regular basis, often in dynamic and profound ways — from childhood to the teen years, teen years to young adult, young adult to middle age, and eventually old age. Changes of location, career, social status. Changes of knowledge and awareness, and acquisition of new skills. Usually, the ordinary changes for us in measured and expected ways.

With chronic pain, as with other disasters, the changes are unexpected and much harder to contend with. The key to countering loss of the ordinary is first understanding your need for it and how you had defined it, and seeing how it has changed, followed by reestablishing some version of it as soon as possible. Explore all the ways in which your new life in chronic pain has changed what was once ordinary, and acknowledge your powerful losses, suffering, and consternation.

Reestablishing the ordinary requires changing your perspective and outlook on life in ways that can offer a new sense of continuity. This includes developing new insights, strategies, skills, and evolved methods of coping. It requires making the choice to create a "new normal" for yourself, one that recreates an "ordinary" you can function in successfully. Understanding how to address the various threats to your needs successfully, as illustrated by the examples in this book, is the key to accomplishing this. As you meet the challenges of chronic pain, you will restore the elements of what contributes to a stable and positive sense of the ordinary. The story of Ralph in the conclusion chapter is an excellent example of this process.

Build Predictability

To contend with unpredictability and limitations, you must first redefine what is predictable and what is doable. Plan for unpredictability and challenge your limitations to whatever extent you can.

Putting some tracking systems in place is a good first step. If you track your day-to-day patterns of pain, functional limitations, and emotional suffering, they become more predictable. This will give you more opportunity to plan, to deal with flare-ups and disruptions, and to minimize their impact on your ability to function predictably.

It helps to learn to be realistic in your expectations. Find ways to make what is possible doable. I have found with many of my clients that once they have taken a problem-solving approach to this challenge, they experience not so much limitations and unpredictability but change — without the usual negative emotional charge. This adjustment can be helped along by being compassionate with yourself about your understandable anger and being able to grieve over your losses.

Most people with chronic pain experience some degree of anger due to all the needs that are threatened by their pain. I had one client who started out directing his anger at all the providers who were disappointing him, and at himself for failing to recover. We worked on turning that energy into changing the way he coped and operated. This included learning new communication and conflict-resolution skills and learning to stop judging himself. The result was much greater progress and predictability with his treatment, and considerably less stress. His example is typical of what happens, and what can happen for you. New opportunities to make your life more predictable occur side by side with loss. If you can embrace them, you will feel more in control and better able to manage your day-to-day life.

Evolve Toward Well-Being

There are many ways to restore a sense of safety and well-being, but almost all require evolving how you operate as a person. This includes developing new coping mechanisms and skills that can produce a level of positive well-being and safety equivalent to the one you had prior to your injury. These are tools of the existential immune system, which are discussed in more detail in chapter 14, "Existential Impacts." They include using your cognitive skills to develop practical ways to create a greater sense of safety in the context of your current limitations. For example, using prosthetics, setting up alert systems to call for help, and developing new skills for self-protection.

Be creative and analytical in developing new ways to have a greater sense of general well-being. This can include embracing your emotions, taking daily doable risks, working on living in the present, being introspective, looking for opportunities to laugh, finding ways to live your personal values, identifying and making use of your individual strengths, being mindful about your thoughts, being vulnerable and open to the protection, support, and assistance of others, and being open and nonjudgmental, insightful, and creative about what will most likely help you. Most importantly, see yourself as wanting and deserving to get what you need to help with your challenges. Know and trust your ability to fight for your secure life and well-being in the world.

Creatively Honor Your Values

Never overlook the importance of values in your life. Values are aspirations we hold that define either who we are or who we want to be in terms of character, behavior, and efforts. Chronic pain can undermine these aspirations, and this can be quite stressful. People fight to support values, even go to war over them. All our decisions are informed by our values, and all our internal conflicts revolve around the dissonance that arises over who we want to be versus who — often driven by necessity — we are.

> "Your ambition to be successful in your career, to be competent, capable, and effective, can be applied to your recovery instead."

Knowing this will help you to understand why the violation of values is so stressful. Understanding the importance that values have in your life will help, as will the many ways you can find to support those values to minimize or eliminate the loss of those aspirations. Let this motivate you to hold true to your values despite any limitations pain might impose upon you. Modify your aspirations to accommodate your current life and its parameters, and you will find that you can still support all your values, even if somewhat differently than before.

Values are not goals but guideposts — choices about what to aspire to and how to live. Rather than being narrowly defined concepts, they are broad notions that can hold a great range of meaning. Take self-reliance, for example: Self-reliance can include knowing when you need to ask for help. Or capableness: If you value being capable, that doesn't mean you can do everything; it might mean you are willing to use prosthetics to achieve higher functioning. If you value ambition, competence, and effectiveness in the context of your career, these values can be applied to your recovery as well. There are more ways than one to define and live by your values. Find ways to be resourceful and creative in how you think about them, honoring the intent behind your chosen values rather than using values as measuring sticks for self-judgment.

Actively Seek Meaning

Understand that there are a multitude of ways to find meaning in the world, to have a sense of purpose, value, and agency. Being meaningful, by definition, is defined as being alive and full of potential.

This means there are many aspects to who you are that are part of your sense of meaning. The solution is to become a seeker after meaning. This may involve learning more about what is important to you. Perhaps you are not currently working at your true purpose in life. Your pain may compel you to decide, finally, what that purpose might be. Think like an entrepreneur. Pain is only the boss if you give it the job. Instead, create a new business for being you that feels meaningful just for you. For instance, I have worked with many injured workers who cannot do physical labor anymore, and instead pursue a new career or start a business. Remember, you get to choose how you experience your reality and what you want to do with it.

Choose Connection

Understand that alienation from people you care about is the result of a colossal misunderstanding of what has happened to you, both by yourself and by others. If you understand this — and hopefully reading this book will enlighten you about it — the likely response will be compassion for yourself and from others. You will be able to access your common bond as humans in the current situation. Remember the elements of your experience that are common to all people: Everyone has experienced physical pain and emotional suffering, some level of significant threat to their needs, or prolonged suffering. If you describe your experience in connection with the experiences of others, they will be much better able to understand what is happening to you. So learn to speak the common language: vulnerability. If your friend has had a toothache and suffered some related emotional loss, try to explain your pain and loss in connection with their experience. Understand that you have nothing to feel embarrassed about or to apologize for. There is no shame in the pain and suffering being human can bring. You are only alone if you don't know how not to be. Let compassion and your willingness to be open and authentic with others help build connection around our shared humanness.

Address Bias and Discrimination from Friends

The many specific solutions to addressing bias and discrimination from providers can be found in part 4, on the treatment environment. When you are addressing bias among family, friends, and acquaintances, remember this: You are the expert on the totality of your condition and the efforts you have made. Assert yourself when others discriminate, articulate the truth, educate and enlighten them, protest if you must. Aim to convert them from detractors to allies. It helps to be open, vulnerable, and proactive with those who misperceive or misunderstand your situation. Share your efforts in recovery. Explain the complexity of your problem. Enlighten them about the scope and impact of collateral damages. Based on this knowledge, help them see the most effective ways they can partner with you and help support your recovery.

Chapter 12

Situational Impacts

I n some way, everything about your lifestyle is likely to be threatened or affected by chronic pain, from your finances and relationships to everyday ways of experiencing yourself and your world. Some of the changes are obvious; others will be less so.

It is hard to let go of the future you had imagined. It is hard to have to change the way you usually operate as a person in most situations. But, as mentioned before, there is opportunity in these challenges. This chapter will help you recognize and then address the wide scope of situational impacts that chronic pain can have on your life.

CHANGED ECONOMIC STATUS

When pain arrives, your financial state is likely to suffer a significant downturn. Mounting medical and other expenses and lost time from work will have a financial impact. You may or may not have financial reserves to deal with this. The complexities of pain treatment add to its cost, and addressing this complexity often involves expensive specialists, tests, treatment modalities, interventions, and surgeries. Even if you're fortunate enough to have medical insurance, many of these expenses are likely not covered.

While you are facing all this complexity, you are also facing the fact that many primary care systems do not routinely support coordinated and integrated chronic pain care. This adds even more to the expense of an already inefficient approach to pain management. Comprehensive pain management programs can be more effective for treatment but can be quite expensive and are often not covered by insurance. To cut costs, many managed care organizations "carve out" portions of comprehensive, integrated programs and send patients to different providers for their various needs, diluting the proven successful outcomes of integrated programs.

It's also possible your pain may cause you to not be able to work. You may have to tap into your savings, investments, or pension plans. You may have to sell your home or downsize. The economic losses from disabling chronic pain are often utterly devastating, and for some may even lead to bankruptcy.

CHANGED SOCIAL STATUS

What we commonly conceptualize as someone's social standing or class is often measured by a combination of education, income, and occupation. Access to resources, privilege, power, and control are often included in these measures, along with attractiveness, physical prowess, health, and wellness.

Social status also has to do with how well a person conforms to social norms, the unwritten rules about acceptable behavior in a group or culture. Every social group has norms that define appropriate behavior. Norms provide order in society. Human beings count on norms to guide and direct our behavior, to provide order and predictability in social relationships, and to make sense of each other's actions. In our society, most people, most of the time, seek to conform to social norms. But what happens when you lose privilege, power and influence, income and occupation, or health and wellness because of chronic pain? You may not be able to conform to social norms. This is a loss, one compounded by the negative views of others caused by bias, ignorance, and misunderstanding of chronic pain. The overall result is social stigma: a decrease in others' estimation of you, and perhaps a decrease of your own estimation of yourself.

In our society, your new identity as a chronic pain patient is not a sign of status. While some may be sympathetic to your suffering, your status as a less-than-functional member of society will diminish your social standing in many circles. Losing a career, being unable to participate in social activities, or exhibiting discomfort around others may also diminish your status. Changes in family function or structure may leave you marginalized at home as well, compounding your loss of status. You may even participate in marginalizing yourself by defining yourself as less worthy.

For many of my clients, loss of social status creates a sense of guilt and shame and a fear of abandonment or excommunication. This contributes to further emotional decline. People who come to believe they no longer deserve help may even stop asking for what they need from providers and others on whom they depend.

LOSS OF SATISFYING SOCIAL ACTIVITIES

Chronic pain can steal you away from enjoying valued activities that connect you with loved ones, friends, and family. It often leaves you feeling isolated, lonely, and rejected. Socializing — in family gatherings, at social and community events, through athletic pursuits or spectator sports — is a hugely important activity for human beings. When it hurts to be active, when you're depressed from unrelenting suffering, or when your energy is drained from fighting pain, it's hard to accept invitations to socialize. It's also hard to commit to planning or attending regularly scheduled events. You never know how you'll feel when it's time to head out the door.

You may quickly tire of having to decline invitations, explain why you must say no, or leave activities early. You may feel embarrassed or fearful of what others will think, worrying that they'll see you as weak or a complainer. At times your pain can leave you so disconnected from life that it's hard to know what else to talk about — but you really don't want to dwell on your suffering, so you don't know how to respond when others ask about your pain. It's hard to articulate how your pain is disabling you, especially if you don't understand the extent of the damage pain has created in your life.

LOSS OF AND/OR DAMAGE TO RELATIONSHIPS

Dealing with chronic pain can be overwhelming. Communicating and staying close to friends and loved ones is critical in helping you cope with that. Unfortunately, just when you need this comfort and closeness the most, the chronic pain experience may create conflict, misunderstandings, and distance. Here are some typical situations:

- You feel angry at anyone who denies the reality or severity of your pain, anxiety, stress, and suffering.
- You're disappointed in others' reactions to your suffering; you feel rejected or judged.
- You feel hurt when others are disappointed by your inability to

perform ordinary tasks and roles, participate in activities, or meet their expectations.

- You are disappointed in yourself over your actual inability to maintain commitments because of your pain.
- Others feel shortchanged or rejected because of your diminished ability to nourish friendships; some friendships end.

Any of these situations can contribute to feelings of marginalization, which may make you more resentful and defensive, and less able to meet the relationship challenges chronic pain presents. Meanwhile,

> "Promising to be with someone 'in sickness and health' is a lot harder to deliver than most people realize."

your experience of suffering from anger, anxiety, or depression may make you feel like an undesirable person to be around. Impatience will build, conflicts will become harder to resolve — over time it becomes easier to deal with social avoidance than social engagement. Others don't know how to react to that and may even feel helpless in dealing with you. Friends, family, even your own physician may pull away, unable to offer attention, empathy, or sympathy.

This kind of situation can snowball as your condition lingers. People living with chronic pain often withdraw from relationships outside their immediate family, which can then lead to estrangement. Loss of friendships and other important relationships is another emotionally disabling aspect of chronic pain.

Chronic pain also changes interactions with spouses, children, and extended family in ways both large and small. For instance, if you are experiencing a pain flare-up or decreased self-esteem, you may rebuff people who reach out to you.

Intimate physical or emotional relations with a partner can be difficult, depending on the source and intensity of the pain and your mutual ability to accommodate your limitations. Your significant other may become depressed in response to the changes in you and their own sense of loss. A partner may also have to take on more household duties and parenting responsibilities as you become less able to function. Money worries due to hospital bills and decreased income can place additional stress on relationships.

For young children, it can be upsetting to see a parent in chronic pain. They may be confused about what's going on and anxious because their future seems uncertain. They may be angry at you for not being as available as you once were. Or they may feel guilty, if they assume they did something to cause your pain, or ashamed, if they're helpless to help you.

Promising to be with someone "in sickness and in health" is a lot harder to deliver than most people realize. When you are suffering from chronic pain, you may have to renegotiate your entire relationship with your significant other and/or your children. Guilt and shame over not being able to be a "good parent" may end up sabotaging your family. Your relationships with them may crumble if adaptations and adjustments are not made successfully. This is especially true when the family or relationship already has problems or is limited in trust and emotional intimacy. Without a commitment to authenticity and a willingness to grow and change, relationships can end in divorce.

You may be disappointed if extended family members are inattentive. Or you may have no family, or none nearby, so you feel as if no one close to you understands the extent of your suffering. The extent of damage to these relationships depends in large measure on your ability to be vulnerable in communicating your needs. But it is likely that any unresolved issues in your family relations will come to the fore when provoked by the needs your pain has created. In this situation, denial, trivialization, and eventual abandonment are common rationalizations for estrangement.

LOST OR CHANGED ROLES

Human beings have many roles in our lives. Some are obvious and some not. Psychological roles — for example, that of a family member who steps in to mitigate conflict with humor — are based on our values and may be almost invisible to those around us. Professional roles are public and often ones we have chosen — dental technician, truck driver, cook, receptionist, carpenter, teacher, soldier. Some roles are defined by birth or circumstance: spouse, parent, or sibling, for instance.

Any and all roles can be targeted by pain. Any role can be undone or significantly compromised. Pain can severely diminish your ability to care for yourself; your role as a self-reliant individual can literally disappear if you can no longer bathe yourself, shave, comb your hair, dress and undress, or even eat without help from others. If your pain interferes with your ability to think clearly and be emotionally grounded, you might not be able to fill the role of the problem solver, the compassionate one, the levelheaded one. You may lose your sense of filling the role of parent if pain makes playing with your children impossible. Or if pain makes lovemaking torturous, you may feel you've lost the role of lover. If you can't work, you cease to be the provider. You may experience guilt over no longer being an able-bodied partner.

All of us expect to help each other out in times of illness or high stress, but those events are usually of short duration. With chronic pain, there may not be an end in sight. And as time goes on, resentment is likely to increase. As you watch loved ones at home and colleagues at work become overburdened by the extra tasks chronic pain necessitates, your own self-esteem and self-worth may plummet, making it more likely that you feel guilty or selfish.

In addition to losing old roles, you will see an increase in new roles, often undesirable ones. You now may be thought of as the promise breaker, the nonproductive one, the unreliable or unpredictable one. In the role of chronic pain patient or disabled person, you may become the person who must fill out numerous forms and complete reports for the Americans with Disabilities Act, state and federal disability insurances, and leaves of absence from work. If your chronic pain resulted from a work-related illness or injury, there is the bureaucratic morass of worker's compensation to navigate, and you must take on the role of claimant. All this leads to filling a filing cabinet and carrying the new role of paper pusher.

REDUCED ABILITY TO WORK

Pain can affect your ability to be productive in every area of your life. You may lose productivity at work, whether because you can't perform at your usual and required standard or because you must miss too many days on the job. This produces high stress and anxiety, which can be amplified if you must take medical leave. You may lose your job, jeopardizing your career and possibly thwarting your future ambitions. You may have to change your pursuits in ways you don't want to. For example, suppose you've been injured after years of work in the trades as a carpenter, plumber, or electrician. You may be compelled to go back to school long after you've forgotten how to be a student, whether or not you have any interest in education or track record of success in what you're now studying. You may have to give up years of accomplishment for an uncertain new endeavor.

At home, productivity relates to all your activities: projects around the house, hobbies you want to pursue, and plans for self-improvement, continuing education, and maintaining physical conditioning and health, to name just a few. All can be thwarted by your chronic pain. Most people's sense of personal value is strongly attached to what they can accomplish and how well they can provide for themselves and others. So the existential cost of lost productivity is often much higher than that measured in dollars.

LOST OR LIMITED OPPORTUNITIES

Chronic pain can limit life's opportunities — and by *opportunities* I'm referring to access to resources: both tangible ones such as food, clothing, and shelter, and intangible ones such as education, health care, careers, relationships, and personal growth. I've had client after client testify to the litany of lost opportunities caused by living with chronic pain.

CHANGED PURSUITS

Chronic pain impacts life pursuits like obstacles in a river: logs here, rock outcroppings there, strong currents, rapids, and even waterfalls. You may get diverted and forced to go down an unexpected path. You may get stuck or have to leave the river altogether and find another way. Pain diverts you from your pursuits and often completely redirects them.

The ambitious pursuit of a career may turn into a desperate struggle to hold onto your job. Just being able to get out of bed in the morning may become your athletic goal. Searching for relief and a cure for your chronic pain can dominate your life as you try a variety of pharmacological, physical, and "alternative" therapies.

Constant pain diminishes your ability to focus, which reduces your ability to find solutions to even relatively mundane problems. You may have difficulty concentrating on simple tasks. Something like a traffic jam, which would mildly annoy most people, can seriously throw off the rhythm of someone who is putting forth every effort just to get through the day.

Pain wears you down, causing you to redirect your energy and your motivation. Instead of seeking activity and connection, all you want is isolation and quiet. You want to simplify your life as much as possible, limiting social contact to reduce stress and decrease the amount of energy you need to spend reacting to your environment. Because pain is exhausting and sleep can help you forget for a while, sleeping may become a more appealing pursuit than living.

Ultimately, chronic pain can change pursuit to avoidance, and the embrace of life to the rejection of engagement.

CHANGED EXPECTATIONS

We all have expectations about both everyday realities and more overarching needs, wants, and goals. Expectations set our mental tone. They influence how we perceive events and how effectively we can respond to challenges. To illustrate: Some of us expect to be able to drive in a large city and have no traffic. When in fact confronted with heavy traffic, these people experience frustration, even rage. A more realistic expectation about traffic would inspire planning and positive distractions, which would minimize negative emotional reactions.

With chronic pain, it may seem as if the only thing you can realistically expect is more pain and suffering. Feeling physically and psychologically normal and healthy, meeting daily needs, achieving goals — all become uncertain. Chronic pain destroys positive expectations and replaces them with negative expectations about all aspects of your future, adding stress to an already overloaded plate.

Understand that chronic pain is like traffic. It interferes with your wanted outcomes. You need to adjust for the reality of how it interferes. Then it will be much easier to have a positive mental tone and to prepare to minimize its impact.

INTERFERENCE WITH LEARNING

Pain is designed to get your attention. And it does that so well you can hardly concentrate on anything else.

Unfortunately, medications to reduce pain can also reduce your ability to focus; some diminish attention and short-term memory too. You may suffer sleep disruption, which further compromises your ability to learn. Chronic pain may cause substance abuse and psychological problems like depression and anxiety. Depression not only affects sleep patterns but can decrease one's motivation and ability to learn new things. Anxiety and anger, so common to chronic pain, disrupt focus and motivation. When chronic pain compromises your mobility, it also makes it difficult to access or use educational resources.

Chronic pain is a teacher. Most people only learn what they cannot know and cannot have. You can learn more than that.

INTERFERENCE WITH NEW AND SATISFYING EXPERIENCES

Chronic pain compromises your ability to have or pursue new and satisfying experiences. Travel, career, education, creativity, relationships, and roles are all compromised or thwarted by the evolution of chronic pain.

As the impacts of chronic pain compound themselves across time, you become less and less likely to consider pursuing new experiences. At some point, you may find that you can't even imagine being able to enjoy them.

RECOVERY: HEALING SITUATIONAL HARM

The positive side of beginning to understand how chronic pain has affected so many aspects of your life is that you can begin to see opportunities for healing that weren't apparent before. The fact that it has changed your day-to-day life gives you a chance to re-envision what life could look like, and to imagine potential improvements in all aspects from finances to relationships. This section addresses, topic by topic, those impacts listed earlier in the chapter.

Make Repairs to Your Lifestyle

Your lifestyle includes many aspects — finances, position, social status, relationships, roles, productivity, opportunity, pursuits, expectations, experiences, activities, and other things that matter to you. To maintain or restore this requires several different efforts. You might feel you have lost the elements that make up your lifestyle or allow you to sustain it. But consider whether they have been truly lost — or just compromised. You may need to find replacements for or restore what's damaged, and to look at the challenge as a problem to be solved rather than as an overwhelming task. If you can be flexible and open to change, if you are willing to redesign and, if necessary, recreate your lifestyle, it likely can be done. If you take this approach, a damaged lifestyle needn't be a call for a teardown and reconstruction of yourself but rather an opportunity, aided by problem-solving and changes to your usual coping methods. Every step you take can further a process of personal transformation.

Mitigate Financial Loss

There are no magic solutions to the potential economic impact from chronic pain. When possible, it's a must to have excellent and comprehensive health insurance, as well as short-term and long-term disability insurance, to absorb and limit direct financial loss. But perhaps more important, regardless of your insurance situation, is the self-awareness made possible by this book and the tools in the appendixes. Many of the most damaging effects of chronic pain are on your ability to function. If these impacts on functioning can be ameliorated or countered, your ability to provide for yourself improves. Thus, there's less economic impact. Truly, your own recovery is the best preventative to bankruptcy.

Reexamine Status as a Value

The extent of impact from loss of status largely depends on how you experience it. While the impacts of chronic pain may disqualify you from a high social status as our culture defines it, you still choose how you define your own standing. If you can limit or marginalize the impacts of chronic pain, reinventing yourself as you do so, you may regain your membership in the groups that matter to you. More importantly, you may seriously question the value — and truth — of social status itself. You might take a hard look at the value of friendships with those who are guided only by social status in their opinion of you.

Reinvent Your Social Network

You can minimize your loss of social activities; the key lies in your willingness to explore and share your vulnerability, your communication and conflict-resolution skills, and your willingness to be flexible and creative. You may not feel comfortable briefing your friends and family about your limitations and emotional state, but it's important to do so. Challenge yourself to find ways to keep engaged with others. Even if you can't be with someone physically, you can phone, email, text, or use social media. Instead of going to a friend's house or out for dinner, invite friends to your home or plan coffee dates via video conference. Let people help you to prepare or clean up after a meal, or even bring you one when needed. Most friends will understand and appreciate knowing how they can help.

Practice vulnerability by enlisting others' aid in helping you make changes in how you interact. Consider new ways to participate with others, and ask them to help you figure it out. Include them in the planning. Ask if they can be tolerant and patient with the unpredictability of your commitments and the constraints you may have to put on your outings. Be forthcoming about your needs for emotional comfort and support. Most people who care about you will feel good about contributing to your well-being. Many would like *any* of your time versus none. But people usually need guidance as to how they can best relate to and help you. There's no shame or guilt in accepting help. Instead, it's a wonderful opportunity to be gracious and grateful.

> "Consider new ways to participate socially with others, and ask them to help you figure it out."

Tend to Your Relationships

Living with chronic pain and staying connected with others depends to a large extent on your ability to live in the truth and adapt to it. It depends on your willingness to acknowledge your limitations to yourself and others and your ability to transform grief and anger over your losses — in short, to reinvent yourself in your relationships.

Here are some strategies to help you stay close to your friends and loved ones:

Find a communication balance. The people you are close to in life need to know how you are feeling. Staying silent will only cause them to feel estranged from you. On the other hand, sharing too much can cause them to feel overwhelmed, helpless, or depressed. Try to find the right balance. Keep in mind that it will be different for each person in your life. You can tell people you'd like to keep them up to date and ask how frequently they would like a check-in, so they can help you find the right balance.

> "Staying connected with others depends largely on your ability to live in the truth and adapt to it."

Discuss your sexuality with your spouse. Chronic pain does not rule out lovemaking, but it can mean that more planning, patience, and creativity are required. Plan encounters that fit into your medication schedule and the ebb and flow of your daily pain. Don't be afraid to experiment with new positions in or approaches to lovemaking and intimacy.

Avoid last-minute cancellations with friends. Don't let chronic pain keep you from interacting with friends altogether. Canceling plans can be disappointing for all concerned, so explain your situation. For example, you can say that you try to accept only the activities you can manage with your pain and that invitations are still welcome, even when you sometimes decline. When meeting in person won't work, consider creative ways of participating — meeting online or by phone, or helping with preparations for events that you may not be able to attend. For example, you may not be able to join in on a cross-country ski outing, but you can meet your friends at the trail end with your famous ginger cookies, and take pictures of cookies coming out of the oven that can be included along with other snapshots from the trip.

Take on manageable household responsibilities. If you find yourself unable to perform certain chores that were once your responsibility, replace them with new tasks that you can perform. This will keep you an active and contributing member of your family. For example, if you can't cook, perhaps you can take on dishwashing; if you can't do your own laundry, maybe you can take over paying the monthly bills.

Ask for help. Giving your loved ones a chance to help you in some way can make them feel closer to you. Often, they want to help but aren't sure how to offer for fear of offending you. If you're having trouble with an activity or chore, ask them to lend a hand. For example, let them help you carry an object that's too heavy for you; let them shop for you if you find that activity too demanding.

Reinvent Your Roles

Obviously, there's profound loss involved when you can no longer fill the roles you used to. But again, there are opportunities to be found. Loss of a role doesn't mean the loss of your value as a person; you are defined not by what you do but by who you are.

Certainly, losses need to be respected and grief acknowledged, but once that happens, energy can be restored and new discoveries made. There might be lateral changes in roles that can offset the losses — shifting from a working parent to become a stay-at-home parent is one example — or opportunities for new roles that could have great value for you and others in your life. Roles where you become more present, or more available, or more useful in general to others. Your condition may require you to develop important interpersonal and intrapersonal skills that can open up new roles in life — to become the good listener, the empathic and compassionate one, the mindful witness.

> "Remember, for all the roles you currently fill, there are many valuable roles you haven't had time to try on."

Chronic pain offers you a unique opportunity. Remember, for all the roles you currently fill, there are many valuable roles you haven't had time to try on. Rather than take on the role of victim or someone defeated by pain, instead look for the means to thrive. Such people become an inspiration to everyone. It's a role available to anyone, and is often the key element to true pain management.

Cultivate Adaptability

Chronic pain can strike at any age and find you in every conceivable work or career situation. Though every solution is dependent on your unique circumstances, the core challenge is the same. It usually involves making a major decision: either finding a way to stay in your job or career, including enlisting the aid of your employer, or reinventing what you do to make a living. How well you can manage the impacts of your pain might determine the extent to which you can maintain what you have.

For instance, in seeking ways to maintain your current career path, you'll need to consider the value of vulnerability and transparent communication. You will need to consider your total skills, experience, and personal traits as they relate to your ability to earn a living. You may decide to reinvent your money-making path. I have many stories of clients going back to school and successfully creating new careers for themselves, and of others who changed professions or started up businesses of their own. Once again, creativity, adaptability, and emotional openness to change will help you respond to this challenge and minimize losses in your work life.

Envision New Opportunities

Chronic pain makes it hard to seize opportunities that can help you achieve the goals you've set. But no matter what your life situation is, there are always opportunities. Opportunity, by definition, means possibility. When you are living with chronic pain, you are likely to experience obstacles on the path to possibility. But you can choose to see each obstacle as a challenge rather than an impediment.

When I had difficulty with board-breaking during my training as a martial artist, my instructor pointed out that I needed to focus my energy on being through and on the other side of the board. This concept can be applied generally: Don't invest your energies in the obstacles in your way. Put your energy over there, on the other side of the obstacle, and you will pass through it much more easily. See your life as you want it to be on the other side of your obstacles. Be your own visionary.

Many of my clients have found positive opportunities in their suffering by finding a path around or through to new and equally rewarding opportunities. In living with their afflictions, actors Michael J. Fox and Christopher Reeve found new opportunities in acting, directing, research, and disability activism. They continue to inspire others to make the best of their lives no matter the obstacles.

Cultivate Willingness to Change

Chronic pain has powerful potential to divert you from your pursuits. It is more likely to succeed if you persist in trying to do things the way you are used to.

In my study of the martial arts, my sensei would often say that for every strike, there is a counter. There is more than one way to follow your pursuits and achieve your goals. Don't get stuck in your preferred way of doing things. You may not like having to ask for the help you need to be successful — unless you appreciate the common humanity it represents. You may need to find ways to better contend with negative thinking, anger, and depression, ways to counter them with more effective coping strategies. For instance, being more open and vulnerable and more comfortable in asking for what you need.

Consider that for most people, the most important thing is wanting to "get things done." You can choose to find a way that works for you. You can choose a path that helps you overcome obstacles but also allows you to remain true to who you are. Be willing to change.

Adjust Expectations

You can avoid having your expectations dashed by chronic pain by understanding the possible conditions you may find yourself in from day to day and designing your expectations realistically. You can become the expert on the patterns of your pain, its flare-ups, and its impact on your functioning. Pain patterns are more predictable than most people realize. By tracking and learning from your patterns, you can begin to plan for them and avoid the frustration of thwarted expectations.

Suppose you have a hard time having to follow Plan B, C, or D when Plan A is the one you want. To avoid unnecessary stress, you need not just your adjustable activity plan (see chapter 6) but an *expectation success plan*. The key to managing the stress of unfulfilled expectations is to plan a way of always expecting what can be achieved, even if that achievement reflects your lowest level of functioning. Based on a range of possibilities, from the most positive state you can hope to be in all the way to the least positive, design your expectations to fit your realities. Trying to do what you cannot will be more stressful than achieving at a lesser level: If deliberate resting becomes your activity, or if you must break up a task into doable bits or get help, this will be less stressful than failing at too big a goal.

Take Care of Your Brain

When pain interferes with your ability to learn, the solution, as with many solutions to chronic pain, comes from your own motivation and commitment to try new behaviors. Practice techniques that enhance concentration and attention, such as meditation or yoga, or cognitively challenging games, such as chess. There are also cognitive remediation programs, commonly used with people with brain injury and Alzheimer's conditions, that you can use for maintaining general brain health. Learning challenges might inspire new study skills, such as finding a tutor to help you learn speed reading or adopting mnemonic techniques to help with retention. Look for a mentor or counselor to support you.

One of the most helpful things you can do is to become less dependent on medications that negatively impact cognition.

Explore New and Satisfying Opportunities

When chronic pain means that some types of new and satisfying experiences are out of your reach, the answer is to adopt a broader view of what you can experience that can still be fulfilling. Consider brainstorming your interests, activities, aptitudes, curiosity, and wishes (whether past or present) to uncover opportunities for doable, new, and satisfying experiences.

Many people haven't fully explored their interests or the things that truly motivate them. When I engage clients in a practice of doing this, they often discover a depth of interest that expands possibilities for meaningful endeavors they can engage in. You may discover a new potential career or some skill that you'd like to develop, like playing the piano or writing. Each time I explore this with my clients, they uncover a long and surprising list of these items. Focus on what matters to you, what you can access and do. Consider how you pace and plan for success in these new endeavors.

Chapter 13

Functional Impacts

Chronic pain damages and affects your ability to function in general, and in specific ways, all resulting in exacerbated pain and less capacity for recovery. It has the potential to undermine your ability to do all of what matters in your life, including enjoying the attributes—emotional, psychological, spiritual, cognitive, and physical—that empower and enable you. Chronic pain can significantly humble or shrink your sense of agency. This chapter aims to help you identify and address the more specific challenges of functional impacts on you as a person from chronic pain.

LIMITED CAPACITY

A clear, functional mind can overcome many physical and emotional limitations, but if you lose your abilities to concentrate, focus, and think, or to remember simple facts and events that happened a short while ago, you may feel increasingly helpless to act. Biologically, pain compromises the regions of the brain that help with the ability to think and concentrate well. Specifically, it compromises a region of the brain known as the lateral occipital complex, which monitors those functions. Most clients I've worked with agree that limitations in the way their mind functions can be even more profound than impacts on physical functioning.

Chronic pain and its accompanying stress may even age the brain faster than normal, shrinking gray matter by a certain percentage each year. One theory on why this happens is that chronic pain forces nerve cells to work overtime.

This is because of the brain's neuroplasticity — meaning the brain's ability to adapt. Physiological changes in the brain happen as a result of our interactions with our environment. Our experiences reorganize neural pathways in the brain that produce long-lasting functional changes. We can see these changes occur when we learn new things or memorize new information. The process can be shaped by experience. As chronic pain continues, then, it may become harder to reverse and less responsive to treatment. With complex regional pain syndrome, chronic pain "rewires" the brain over time and can cause you to feel pain where there is no injury.

Chronic pain may also undermine your existential capacity — your ability to "be" in the world and to have a will to live and to thrive. This is your essential motivation; it includes your capacity to decide and choose and not just react. Chronic pain may thus weaken your capacity to deal with threats to your needs. Given the multiple crises and ongoing stressors you experience with chronic pain, it's like facing a war on too many fronts; it limits your capacity for managing stress. It's hard to have positive experiences and feel happy feelings when chronic pain brings so many negative emotions. Ultimately, your overall capacity to manage pain may seem to be diminishing in a downward spiral.

REDUCED COMPETENCE

Competence is a way of being. It's often thought of as a relatively permanent quality of personality that's valued by an individual and their community. Competence is seen not simply as a skill but as a virtue: it has personal, social, moral, and intellectual characteristics.

A loss of competence equates to a loss of capability; it makes you feel insecure in handling the tasks that life presents. On a practical level, competence is knowing you can consistently perform the tasks you need to perform; when you feel unable to do that, you feel incompetent. For most people, level of competency is an important aspect of how you see yourself and who you are — a part of your identity.

There's an important distinction between *competence* (or capability) and *competencies* (which are specific skill sets). Competencies describe outcomes of achievement and involve specific knowledge, attributes, and behaviors necessary to fulfill specific tasks. Competence is a more general quality, but it is no less powerful. When its associated physical and emotional states interfere with your potential to perform, chronic pain can trash your competence.

UNDERMINED ABILITY FOR SELF-CARE

Self-care is each person's personal responsibility. Most of us take our ability for self-care for granted, though we may practice it with varying degrees of commitment and success. However, chronic pain can undermine and make good self-care difficult, if not impossible.

Self-care includes all activities of daily living, including bathing, defecating and urinating, preparing meals, cleaning house, doing laundry, and personal grooming. It includes all the health decisions you make for yourself to ensure you are physically and mentally fit. This includes exercising, eating well, and practicing good hygiene. It also includes your effort to prevent ill health or harm by avoiding hazards such as smoking, drinking, and unsafe driving. Self-care also means taking care of minor ailments and long-term conditions and following recommended treatments. It involves maintaining personal safety and emotional satisfaction.

When capacity for self-care is undermined by chronic pain, adjustments in behavior and outlook can be a successful counter, as described further in the Recovery section.

INCREASED DEPENDENCE

Dependence and independence can be thought of as a continuum of self-reliance. At one end of this spectrum is total reliance (complete dependence) upon a partner, family member, friend, or caregiver. At the far extreme, this equates to living like an infant or young child, where someone else must provide you with a place to live, feed you and clothe you, take care of your bodily needs, and define your role in the family unit or wider community.

At the other end of this spectrum is total self-reliance (complete independence). This means you provide your own food and shelter, roles and relationships, productivity and opportunities.

Your personality and the situation at hand will determine your comfort level with receiving help in general, and which kinds of help. Associations with dependence from childhood will also affect your reactions to this as an adult. While you might have very positive associations with being safe and dependent as a child, as an adult you could still have a lot of trouble being helped by others — especially with deep self-care like toileting. On the other hand, you might have very negative associations with being dependent as a child — say if you were dependent on caregivers who were neglectful or abusive. This might make you resistant to receiving help as an adult in any way. You may not like being in someone else's care, or you might be fearful of being disappointed again. On the other hand, you might try to be open to receiving what you need and love (finally) being able to be cared for.

> "Receiving help will either magnify your sense of loss and suffering or be empowering and reassuring."

In other words, your personal history matters in how able you are to get your needs met. How you experience receiving help in the present, when chronic pain diminishes your self-reliance, will either magnify your sense of loss and suffering or be empowering and reassuring. Fear of becoming too dependent may cloud your perceptions. If you don't have childhood associations that suggest a loss of autonomy or a lack of safety when receiving help, it will be easier for you to accept assistance now.

For instance, your partner may offer to help you cook supper and communicate that they enjoy working in the kitchen with you. Perhaps this leads to your partner feeling helpful to you, and you feeling cared for, loved, and supported. In this event, you can accept the help you need, and this kind of sharing can even deepen your relationship.

But what if, instead, your partner's offer to help cook makes you suspect they think less of you or are resentful of your need for help? This can make you feel shamed and diminished, or even controlled or marginalized. You may not receive this offer of help positively, even though your partner's intention was to support you during trying circumstances, not to cause you grief and harm. You may even hurt your partner's feelings when you say, "I don't want your help." Your orientation toward your need for others and your associations with these needs can either support you getting needed help or add to barriers to recovery.

Also, sometimes it's hard for others to know how long you need to rely on their help, or when the need for it has passed. It's like knowing when to let go of a child's two wheeler, hoping they won't fall.

REDUCED PROBLEM-SOLVING ABILITIES

Chronic pain taxes and can even overwhelm your problem-solving abilities. Your ability to envision solutions deteriorates when you can't think or analyze or synthesize data. Due to all the disruptions caused by your pain, solving difficult problems may become unmanageable, no matter how hard you try. In this situation, you may have experiences like these:

- If someone opposes you, you find it hard to stick to your aims and get what you want.

- Unexpected events undermine your confidence; you have lost your sense of resourcefulness in handling unforeseen situations.
- It's hard to remain calm or think clearly when issues arise, because you can no longer rely on your problem-solving abilities.

REDUCED ABILITY TO COPE

A state of stress is created when important needs are threatened. Unfortunately, chronic pain rates high as a threat while simultaneously diminishing your ability to cope with the resulting stress.

Coping is the successful — or at least adequate — ability to handle something difficult in response to whatever threatens your needs. Coping skills are the behaviors, thoughts, and emotions that help you maintain your mental health and your physical and emotional well-being. Some coping styles are more effective than others, depending on the person involved and the nature of the stressful situation.

RECOVERY: COUNTERING FUNCTIONAL IMPACTS

Chronic pain gives all strategies new meaning and importance. *Active* strategies have much greater potential to help than coping mechanisms, which don't move you toward your goal of recovery. At times, you may find yourself severely challenged by the sheer scope and intensity of the stressors that you face. But if you make a conscious practice of using active coping strategies, they will become habits that serve you well.

Some strategies may seem daunting to you personally, but they can be very helpful and produce lasting counters to your functional limitations. These are the commonalities: Being practical and using your common sense and intelligence. Being analytical, organized, disciplined, creative, and resourceful in managing your time and tasks. Understanding the realities of the negative impacts your pain has caused, and being patient and realistic in your expectations and compassionate with yourself. Being sure to honor and value your efforts and your determination to reach your goals. Using techniques like meditation, relaxation, physical recreation, and humor to manage your energy, stamina, fortitude, and focus. Seeking support and help whenever you need it to empower your recovery. Finding inspiration and purpose in your efforts to overcome your limitations. Respecting your emotional pain and vulnerability without self-doubt or shame. And appreciating your value and importance as a person.

Cultivate Attitude

What can you do when pain has reduced your capacities and capabilities? As countless clients have taught me, the answer is straightforward: What's been lost can be regained. Capacity and capability can be enhanced and developed. There are activities and strategies to counter this erosion, which you can purposefully choose to engage yourself in.

> "The answer is straightfoward: What's been lost can be regained."

Here are some examples. People with ADD (attention deficit disorder) can increase their ability to attend, focus, and concentrate through various disciplines and cognitive practices. People who use wheelchairs or other assistive devices employ technology to retain their ability to function. People who are vision- or hearing-impaired have many means to exercise their capacities and capabilities. A person who loses a limb may learn to use a prosthetic successfully.

Whenever your pain imposes on your capacities and capabilities, ask yourself: What is the "prosthetic" for this?

Find Competency Workarounds

You do not necessarily lose competence with chronic pain. There are many ways to achieve competence by carrying out tasks differently than you used to. However, you may have to figure out ways to manage pain's impacts and interference with your workarounds.

Two simple examples of workarounds are tying your shoelaces sitting down instead of bending over (for back pain or balance challenges) and dictating the bulk of your communications instead of typing them (for hand pain or focusing problems). With simple adjustments like these, you can work to reestablish task competence. You will be able to do this if you don't stifle yourself with anxious and angry concern over what's been lost.

It's important to make a realistic plan of action for yourself that includes two things. One is an accurate understanding of the limitations imposed by your pain. The second is an assessment of the skills, knowledge, attitude, and behaviors that you'll need to develop — or modify — to accomplish the task. Be willing to adapt to the ever-changing (and often unpredictable) circumstances of your pain condition. As Bruce Lee, the famous martial artist, suggested, learn to "be like water."

You can continue to feel like a competent person by honoring your intention in life, not solely the outcomes of your activities. By basing your perception of yourself on who you are, not what you can do. Be competent at committing and recommitting to what you want to do well until you get it done. Don't get trapped in the idea that there's only one way to do it.

Let Self-Care Become a Team Task

The greatest barrier to restoring your ability to care for yourself is *not* chronic pain. It is the reluctance to rely on others and to be emotionally vulnerable. Making modifications and accepting help are the keys to overcoming your challenges to self-care.

To begin to rely on others requires an understanding that there are some things you just cannot do by yourself. That this is not a call for guilt, shame, or self-judgment. Be aware that others in your life often want to find ways to be helpful; they may be much more willing to help if you ask. Chronic pain causes a great deal of emotional suffering, which is something everyone understands. Just as we lean on others when we lose someone, and come together to share the burden, the emotional burden of your suffering can be shared.

Working with others to help you with self-care restores what has been lost. *The restoration of functioning is more important than the means you use to accomplish it.* It is through problem-solving and practicality that you can restore your sense of self-sufficiency and self-care, not through rigid and limited ideas of what it means to be self-reliant.

Return Gradually to More Self-Reliance

A willingness to accept help when you need it is an important part of self-reliance, but one to be balanced and considered in context of the need for agency and independence. Not accepting needed assistance can be unhealthy and self-diminishing in its own way, but so can overdependency. When possible, it's important to reclaim a portion of your independence as soon as you can. If you're willing to change your standards for performing routine tasks, you may be able to return to doing them again on your own, and in your own way, much more quickly. Be flexible in the ways you view dependence and self-reliance. What's most important is how an action makes you feel, not the specifics of how you do it.

Go into Problem-Solving Mode

Most people are unaware that chronic pain can modify a person's entire way of getting their needs met, in a manner that can weaken typical problem-solving strategies and skills. This difficulty can be countered from two different angles. First, you can maintain a higher level of problem-solving skill by using the suggestions described in this book to minimize and marginalize the impacts of chronic pain. Second, you can lean into the many books and resources available about problem-solving methods. Here are some examples of techniques:

- Brainstorming with others, whether professionals or supportive friends, to identify solutions. This activity produces ideas that you can then combine or develop until an optimal solution is found.
- Breaking down large, complex problems into smaller, more easily solvable, "bite-size" problems.
- Considering as many possibilities as you can for the solution to a problem and systematically trying them out.
- Being creative and innovative.
- Taking defined steps toward your goals — doing as much as you can to start with — to help reveal the rest of the solution.
- Trying to put things together in a new way to reveal new solutions.
- Looking at a problem as part of a combination of many elements and variables. For instance, seek a treatment provider with a better understanding of how the challenges of managed care (see part 4, on the treatment experience) can undermine recovery.
- Simplifying a problem into one for which solutions exist. For instance, you can't be cured of your pain, but you can learn many ways of managing it that can increase your functioning.
- Using existing ideas or adapting existing solutions to similar problems. For example, use the concept of physical prosthetics to help with the emotional impact from your pain, like the way an AA sponsor and meetings support recovery from alcoholism.
- Defining the heart of the problem before you seek a solution. For instance, following the concepts in this book, define the collateral damages that chronic pain causes in your life.
- Testing possible solutions until you find the right one.
- Using time- and practice-tested solutions that have been consistently successful with similar problems.
- Patting yourself on the back for every gain.

Adopt Specific Coping Strategies

All coping strategies base their value on the extent to which they reduce the threats to your needs. Coping can be either active or avoidant. Avoidant coping is characterized by consciously or unconsciously ignoring issues;

it often leads to behaviors that aid in the denial of the problem (e.g., drinking, sleeping, isolating). These ineffective coping mechanisms, also referred to as maladaptive coping, are often chosen unconsciously. And they are usually counterproductive.

> "Make a conscious practice of using active coping strategies."

Avoidant strategies may appear to make sense on the surface, and often they can be at least temporarily helpful, but eventually the downside outweighs any benefits. Here are some typical avoidant coping behaviors for chronic pain:

- Keeping yourself distracted.
- Pushing through it.
- Staying busy and often doing too much.
- *Not* doing much; trying to avoid people and situations
- Sleeping a lot.
- Trying to wish your pain away or pretend it isn't happening.
- Obsessing or constantly complaining about your pain, believing that will help.
- Stuffing down your feelings about it, believing *that* will help.
- Excessive drinking or harmful drugs.
- Getting down on yourself, blaming others for your suffering, or pushing people away with irritability and anger.

Unlike avoidant coping, *active* coping strategies involve an awareness of the stressor, followed by attempts to reduce its negative consequences. Some approaches focus on ways to tackle the issues and reduce the stress around a given situation. Other approaches focus on ways to nurture emotional health during the stressful period. These strategies may be challenged by your pain and suffering, but they can be very helpful and produce long-lasting gains. Here are some typical active coping strategies for chronic pain:

- Being practical and using your common sense and intelligence to overcome your challenges.
- Being analytical, organized, disciplined, creative, and resourceful in managing your time and tasks.
- Understanding the realities of the negative impacts that your pain has caused.
- Being patient and realistic in your expectations, and compassionate with yourself.
- Honoring and valuing your efforts and determination to reach your goals.

- Using meditation, relaxation, physical recreation, and humor.
- Managing your energy with stamina, fortitude, and focus, in a way that will do the most good.
- Seeking support and help whenever you need it, if it empowers your recovery.
- Finding inspiration and purpose in your efforts to overcome your limitations.
- Respecting your emotional pain and vulnerability, without self-doubt or shame.
- Appreciating your value and importance as a person.

Chronic pain gives all these strategies new meaning and importance. But in general, avoidant strategies are maladaptive. When used routinely against chronic pain, they can become toxic and fail to bring you toward your goal of recovery.

Active strategies have much greater potential to help and are better suited to long-term solutions and recovery. At times, you may find yourself severely challenged by the sheer scope and intensity of the stressors that you face. But if you make a conscious practice of using active coping strategies, they will become habits that serve you well.

Chapter 14

Existential Impacts

Pain affects what does and doesn't happen in your day-to-day life — your existence. It affects how you think and feel about what's happening. This creates changes in your internal experience: your personal responses to what is happening in your life. How you think and feel about these changes may add to the negative impacts of your pain. You may or may not be aware of the impacts, the life changes, covered in this chapter. But any of these impacts you experience — aware or not — become additional elements of collateral damage that you will want to attend to and counter. If you don't address these types of impacts, they can add substantially to your stress, pain, and sense of loss, undermining your efforts toward recovery.

LIFE INTERFERENCE

Here's a common complaint among people with chronic pain: "I can't have the life I wanted. This is not how I imagined my life would be."

Here are some examples: An eighteen-year-old high school basketball player never has the chance to go pro because of a back injury. A college graduate who planned on law school cannot score high enough on the entrance exam because of cognitive impairment from her pain medications. After apprenticing for ten years, a carpenter has a job injury that stops a career he'd wanted ever since a childhood helping his father build things.

Chronic pain interferes not just with careers but also with roles and responsibilities and even your sense of self, or identity. Some people with chronic pain give up on marriage or having children. Some shy away from any activity that requires them to perform consistently. Many experience constant frustration, worry, disruption, and obstacles to their goals.

LOSS OF PRIVACY

Losing control, losing the sanctity of one's private self, is one of the most prevalent fears people have. Chronic pain increases this fear because of the possibility that basic physical needs might be met only with the aid of others. Pain may also make you feel emotionally overwhelmed and fearful of showing feelings you may be ashamed of. Your physical and emotional privacy may feel at stake. This may lead you to feel uncomfortably vulnerable and dependent on others, which in turn may affect how you feel about yourself.

Loss of privacy or physical independence can lead to negative thoughts and behaviors, excessive anxiety, anger, and eventually depression.

INCREASED VULNERABILITY

Persistent pain and suffering can take away much of your sense of control, your feeling of security, even your feeling of physical and emotional safety. You may lose many of the things that have made you feel comfortable with yourself and your life. You may lose your ability to insulate yourself from hard realities and negative reactions. All the ways you used to be able to manage your life can collapse under the sheer volume of impacts from your pain. Your sense of personal power may come to feel like mist in a strong breeze. Eventually you may be concerned that you are losing the ability to operate autonomously.

You may also become less capable of protecting your own interests. For example, if you feel compromised both cognitively and emotionally, you may have trouble providing independent judgment, decision-making, and accurate assessments of important situations. This can apply to the realm of medical treatment as well as other life decisions. You may be or feel yourself to be susceptible to misperceiving the benefits and risks of treatment as well as of other financial and life decisions. You may begin to see yourself, in a negative sense, as becoming part of a population requiring special protections or control. This may further undermine your sense of control and security, even though the efforts to serve these groups are meant to help.

You may perceive your situation as one that makes you inferior in some way, especially if you allow it to be a threat to your self image or ego. A negative reaction to the sense of insecurity prompted by your pain may make you feel your emotional state is unstable. This sense of insecurity, vulnerability, and loss of control can significantly undermine anybody's positivity and happiness, and you may not be comfortable with expressing your negative emotions openly. This may cause you shame or guilt. Setbacks in any aspect of your sense of safety as a person can eventually weaken your psychological and emotional resilience.

REDUCED CONFIDENCE

Chronic pain erodes confidence. One of my clients, Marie, explains it this way: "It's hard to remember exactly when it happened. Somewhere along the way I realized that I'd lost my confidence. Not just in terms of my ability to conquer my pain, but in everything else. The person who could do anything was gone. Things that had previously seemed nothing more than little challenges suddenly became evidence of what I could not do. I was terrified."

Marie had taken her confidence for granted since grade school. She believed she could handle anything and everything: jobs, relationships, adventures, moving across country, any and all other changes in her life. When her confidence disappeared, she felt lost in unfamiliar territory, vulnerable and helpless.

The fact that her confidence disappeared gradually compounded its impact; by the time she fully noticed it, she was shocked into withdrawing into herself and shutting the world out. She stopped going out with friends and no longer invited them to her place. She became afraid to leave her home. She felt exposed and undesirable. This was one of the worst experiences caused by her pain. The bottom dropped out of her self-esteem. She couldn't fake it: No matter how hard she tried to appear like her old self, Marie felt like she'd experienced the death of the person she had been. All that remained was the shell.

DAMAGE TO CREATIVITY

Pain and creativity, are commonly believed to go hand in hand, like madness and genius. It's said that painful events spark creativity, or that great losses inspire poetry. We imagine musicians writing their best music when at an all-time low, or artists painting their best creations when severely depressed.

It's true that some of the most famous creative works have been accomplished when the artist was suffering, but here is the real question: Does pain make people creative? Or is creativity a way to deal with pain?

Regardless of which philosophical position you take, you should know pain can easily *interfere* with the creative process. There is a point at which physical pain becomes so unbearable that you can think of nothing but the pain. If you lived a creative life before your pain hit, this inability to attend to your creative expression will produce a great sense of loss. More importantly, it is likely to sap your ability to seek novel, diverse, and potent solutions to mastering your pain.

> "Here is the real question: Does pain make people creative? Or is creativity a way to deal with pain?"

LOSS OF IDENTITY

Chronic pain easily strips away layers of what we think of as our identity. If you identify with your job, and pain prevents you from working, then a major piece of your identity disappears. If you identify with your marriage, and pain contributes to divorce, then a major piece of your identity disappears along with your partner. Chronic pain can change everything about the way you once defined yourself and the way you interact with the rest of the world. The person you have become now feels flimsy and fragile, filled with new limitations and easily reached breaking points. With your foundation for your sense of self made unstable, your coping skills crumble.

When Alfred was twenty-five, he thought he knew who he was. He was quite sure of himself after an academic path of earning a PhD in physics and doing postdoctoral research in Europe. He expected to gain a post as a lecturer by age thirty and be a professor by forty. His parents were proud. Alfred was respected by his colleagues and had a wonderful girlfriend and many good friends. Outside of work and relationships, he enjoyed an active athletic life.

All this ended abruptly when a car accident damaged his back. At first, his pain seemed a temporary intrusion into his existence. He still held onto his identity as a scientist and imagined he would return to his career in physics. However, within a year, he'd lost his girlfriend and realized he would not be returning to his work. His identity was falling away as a social, professional, and athletic person.

All-encompassing losses like these can feel very much as if the you that you know is dying. What seemed like essential parts of your life disappear.

This can be frightening, and your reaction may be to embrace a new, less positive identity. In the face of severe or chronic pain, some people begin to identify themselves with the diagnosis itself—a chronic pain patient, not a person with chronic pain. Once pain becomes your new mask, it can be hard to drop. It becomes an obstacle to your recovery. Hiding behind the mask of pain is a poor substitute for being you.

LOSS OF SELF-IMAGE

Self-image is fundamentally social in nature, meaning that your image of yourself is reflected by those around you. So, you see yourself in the way others around you mirror back who you are. As your life changes with the passing of years, so does your self-image. But pain may force you, prematurely, to relinquish your current self-image. If this happens before you have developed a new self-image that you value, your suffering can be fundamental.

For those who restrict their lives, live in isolation as much as possible, and feel like a burden to others, the social reflections that supported their former positive self-image are simply no longer available. As the pain continues, these losses accumulate. They may include loss of productivity, resulting in financial crises, family strain, and stigma.

Cultural values such as independence, hard work, and individual responsibility, when compromised, contribute to your sense of loss, too, as you lose the ability to perform in the way you once did. Over time, all these losses result in a diminished self-concept and negative changes to your self-image. You may see your dependency reflecting negatively on you. You may feel you must return to your "normal" life to maintain a positive self-image. Loss of positive self-image can diminish compassionate responses from yourself, and possibly from others as well.

LOSS OF SELF-WORTH

Self-worth may plummet because of chronic pain and its impact on your ability to perform conventional tasks and meet typical social obligations. If you tend to be self-critical and downplay or ignore your innate qualities, you may begin to use negative words to describe yourself. This can multiply your sadness, depression, anxiety, anger, shame, guilt, and relationship problems.

If you feel diminished, you may begin to tolerate all sorts of unreasonable behavior from your partner or others. Or you may feel unreasonably angry and bully others. Your diminished self-worth may make you doubt all your abilities and be even more avoidant of the challenges your pain presents. Or, conversely, you may try too hard to accomplish tasks, running the risk of more self-diminishing failures.

Chronic pain makes it easy to be afraid that you will be judged negatively by others. If your loss of self-worth makes you feel more self-conscious, you may begin looking for signs that people don't like you or are talking about you negatively. You may become so down on yourself that you begin to abuse yourself by drinking too much, overusing drugs, developing an eating disorder, or making attempts at suicide.

Just when you most need positive reflections from others about your worth, you may be withdrawing from old friends and social groups. This makes you lonelier and makes it easier for your self-assessments to spiral downward.

INCREASED GUILT AND SHAME

Unfortunately, when you're suffering with chronic pain, feelings of guilt and shame are not uncommon. There are two parts of your life where this may show up: with others and toward yourself. These two experiences are different, though often intertwined. Guilt is a painful feeling of regret and responsibility for one's actions (or inactions). Guilt is usually generated by actions that inflict suffering, intentionally or unintentionally, upon another person. Shame is a painful feeling about oneself as a person.

For example, I once said something hurtful to someone at a dinner party. On some level, I knew it was intentional. Afterward, I felt guilty about my actions, especially when I saw how much harm I had caused. More distressingly, I also felt shame that I was the sort of person who would behave that way. Even though I apologized, the damage to my self-esteem lingered. It was quite stressful.

Like many people with chronic pain, you may feel guilty and ashamed about all that you need to do but cannot do without help. You may believe that others interpret your limits as something shameful as well. This will make it hard to even ask for help. Another problem is the frequent confusion and misunderstanding that you and others may have about the impacts of your pain — as described throughout this book.

For example, if you believe you're not trying hard enough to recover, it may undermine your efforts to get what you need from others. Others may not see what you need because they may think that you're dramatizing your pain. If you feel undeserving of help, you may want others to "just know" what you need. If you can't ask or others don't offer, you may believe that they think you don't deserve help! This can lead to plenty of awkward moments where you and others end up in growing frustration and anger. These situations increase your sense of helplessness, guilt, and shame.

Guilt and shame impede growth, change, curiosity, and creativity. In other words, they undermine a positive sense of self. They make you feel diminished and fearful of being exposed, which can lead to withdrawing from relationships. They make you feel powerless to act.

> **"Guilt and shame impede growth, change, curiosity, and creativity."**

Guilt and shame can control your behavior by restraining self-expression and even inhibiting the expression of your emotions. Guilt and shame also tend to make people feel humiliated, which can trigger a desire to retaliate. People feeling deeply ashamed can be self-destructive, indirectly aggressive, or malevolent. They may cover up or compensate for feelings of shame with attitudes of contempt, superiority, domineering or bullying, self-deprecation, or obsessive perfectionism. These feelings can even contribute to the development of mental illness, including addictive disorders, eating disorders, phobias, and sexual dysfunction.

LOSS OF SELF-CONTINUITY

Personal continuity means *persistence in being yourself*— uninterrupted connection concerning you, your life, your personality. Personal continuity is a central feature of identity, and losing it is one of chronic pain's most powerful impacts.

Self-continuity is developed over the course of your life as the organizational structure for how you define yourself. It is your constant, your foundation for daily living. What happens, then, when chronic pain redefines the typical operations of the self? What happens when the pain makes everything about you inconsistent with your core self-concept? Or when pain makes your present self-concept unsustainable and incompatible with the self you thought you knew? This is a subtle but powerful contributor to the negative impacts from your pain. It produces stress at an existential level.

LOSS OF PURPOSE

Chronic pain interferes with and can destroy your sense of meaning, purpose, and power in life.

People have a fundamental drive to find meaning or purpose in life. Having a sense of purpose, whether simple or grand, gives meaning to life and strengthens self-worth. Feeling adrift in that regard, losing a sense of purpose, is one of the greatest harms from chronic pain. People want to matter, to feel a sense of mission, power, and anticipation about life. The absence of these things can lead to confusion, to an inability to commit, and to a waste of time, energy, and resources. The feeling of "just surviving" in the face of chronic pain can leave you asking the existential question, *Is this it?* With no sense of mission or purpose, you may lose hope for a future that can pull you back to an active life.

Purpose is critical to community also, and inseparable from a sense of belonging; when you have one, you have the other. A life filled with positive and enduring relationships nurtures a sense of purpose and alignment with others. Without this, you can feel increasingly alienated and marginalized, believing there must be more to life but feeling powerless to find it. The real cost of not mastering your relationship to chronic pain is the resulting perception that you are leading a shallow and insignificant life, focused only on an unending battle with your pain.

LOSS OF THE PERSON YOU WANT TO BE

Who are you and who do you want to be? These are existential questions on which most people place a great deal of importance. The answers are a large part of your identity and your desires and aspirations in life. It's possible that before your chronic pain, you were clear on who you are or want to be. Or perhaps you were drifting through life, letting the things that happen to you determine who you are. But when chronic pain hits, it may feel as if you have no choice but to follow where it takes you — which may be very radically, negatively different from your pre-pain expectations. This is a significant existential injury that can add considerably to stress, frustration, anxiety, and sense of loss.

REDUCED PLEASURE AND SATISFACTION IN LIFE

Chronic pain robs you of pleasure and satisfaction in life by damaging, interfering with, or destroying much of what is important to you. As humans, most of us desire to be pleased and satisfied with our lives. It is a central need. It's hard to be pleased and satisfied when your ability to function, mood, self-esteem, well-being, and overall happiness are constantly at risk. Chronic pain makes it hard not to focus on the negative. And focusing on the negative breeds dissatisfaction, displeasure, and more dysfunction, which brings less and less pleasure and satisfaction.

UNDERMINED CAPACITY TO ENJOY LIFE

Chronic pain wears down your capacity to enjoy life, a capacity that is dependent upon your emotional well-being. Enjoying life is not necessarily the absence of negative emotions. It's more about a balance between negative feelings and positive ones. The way most of us generate a positive sense of well-being is by being able to function in society, meet the demands of everyday life, experience good mental health, and recover effectively from illness, change, or misfortune. As we know, all these capacities are threatened by the sheer volume of collateral damages caused by chronic pain. You are likely to respond with anxiety and anger. In my experience with hundreds of people suffering from chronic pain, these negative emotions are usually just as damaging as — or even more damaging than — the physical injury that caused the pain.

RECOVERY: COUNTERING EXISTENTIAL LOSSES

Countering your existential losses involves actively and consciously taking back some control over your personal responses to your existing and potential damages. This section outlines how to address each of the aspects of existential loss, now that they have been brought to your attention.

Invest in Understanding

Chronic pain interferes with life. By understanding the existential aspects of your life and how chronic pain affects them, you can learn to minimize, mitigate, or marginalize the collateral damages. Recovery requires a fundamental understanding of what tools are available, especially those you have within yourself, and how to apply them. In doing so, you'll not only be better able to manage pain and thrive, you'll also discover many inner strengths you may not have been aware of. It is more empowering to look for possibilities and opportunities in yourself and in life all around you than to see yourself as engaged in a war with the interferences from chronic pain. Invest in finding and learning strategies that tap into your potential.

Counter Private Losses with Awareness

With chronic pain, potentially nothing is private anymore — not about your physical self, not about your emotional self. Much of the stress associated with loss of privacy relates to your comfort with yourself and with your vulnerability as a human. If you are uncomfortable being helped or expressing your feelings, if you are self-conscious or unduly concerned about what others may think of you, the situation becomes more stressful. But here's one helpful thing to remember: Stress is not in the situation itself; it is in your perception of what is happening. And your perception can change.

> "Having human needs is not shameful. You might work at reminding yourself of this each day."

Perception is based on awareness. If you are compassionate with yourself, your awareness can put your loss of privacy in the context of what has happened to you. Then you see your needs not as an embarrassment or a defeat but as part of a plan to help you recover and thrive.

Having human needs is not shameful. You might work at reminding yourself of this each day. The more comfortable you are with yourself, the more you respect your own needs and yourself, the more deserving you will feel of receiving help. Work on "being okay" as a person, despite your pain. Even if you are understandably regretful that you need help, be gracious to yourself and others in receiving it. The more normal it becomes to share your feelings, and even your private life, the less traumatic these events will be. This is very simple but profoundly true: The more you can acknowledge and embrace the changes your pain has caused, the more you reduce their emotional harm.

Recognize the Limits of Knowing

The loss of control, insecurity, and growing sense of vulnerability caused by chronic pain causes significant stress. The first thing you can do to bring this stress under control is show respect and compassion for your situation and your feelings, and to more realistically manage expectations about what is and isn't certain. When you give up unrealistic expectations, you limit the damage caused by your loss of control. By acknowledging the current negative realities of your situation, as tough as that may be, you will also begin to see new possibilities and new, more reassuring expectations.

Recognize that your pain-related future, by its very nature, is uncertain. Even though it is painful and frightening, try to see things as they really are. Let go of your anxiety and state of dread by accepting personal responsibility — not for the future, but for all the choices you freely make in the here and now. You get to choose how you respond to the things that are presented.

But what is in your control and what is not? Mental attitudes such as desires, hopes, wishes, and preferences are generally in your control even when external things are not. Yes, you do have to work within the limits of probability to make rational choices. Yes, you must make choices based on the evidence before you. Yes, this is exactly where your freedom over the future lies: seeing the truth in your current situation at the greatest depth and breadth that you can. This can build a bridge of certitude across the divide between now and what happens to you next.

By working from a realistic understanding of your current circumstances, you're likely to make progress in the direction you're shooting for. Vulnerability about negative realities and your normal human reactions to them, once embraced, can serve you well in feeling more secure in your life.

> "Seeing the truth in your current situation can build a bridge of certitude across the divide between now and what happens to you next."

Develop a Deeper Confidence

Chronic pain can threaten to unravel your world and challenge every confidence you have about your abilities and standing in life. Yet it also presents you with the opportunity to prevent this.

For most people, confidence is based on their ability to do many things with competence. This involves knowledge and skills, both of which are very important in helping you get your needs met. However, there is a deeper source that supports confidence and is critical in dealing with life-changing events. This deeper confidence comes from discovering your true self, your innate potential, the essence of who you really are without any props. *It is based not on what you have mastered, but on your ability to master whatever you need to.*

Loss of confidence can be a challenge to you to delve deeper into your innate potential, your true nature. Daring to go inward will produce an unshakable new confidence — based on your potential, not your present circumstances. This new confidence has nothing to do with the outer manifestations of your supposed self. It has everything to do with know-ing who and what you truly are. Developing this confidence involves a positive process of self-discovery; it's an opportunity for a journey into mastery.

There are many challenges in life; chronic pain is just one. In all significant life achievements, in our striving to go beyond our own sense of limit, we are often pleasantly surprised to find we can do more, achieve more, and have more. The kind of confidence we achieve in this effort is far more permanent and always adds to a sense of our own value.

Use, Don't Lose, Your Creativity

Creativity can mitigate pain, and pain can inspire creativity. Creativity is energizing. What you think about and how you think can change how you experience pain.

Childbirth is an example of this phenomenon. It's well known that when you concentrate on something other than your pain, or when you understand it that it is short term, you are generally able to cope with it better. The pain of childbirth, for instance, becomes more bearable for some by focusing on the fact that it is temporary, or on the opportunities that bringing forth a brand-new human being can present, including opportunities for personal growth and inspiration.

> **"The creative process can prevent the pain signal from reaching your central nervous system."**

Using the creative process doesn't just distract your mind; it can prevent the pain signal from reaching your central nervous system and replace it with a signal that promotes positive change in that system, which creates a greater strength to cope. Music and other arts such as painting, sculpting, sketching, dancing, acting, and so on will focus attention away from pain and be empowering and energizing. Creative therapies have been introduced into many hospital and community settings to help people embrace and transform their chronic suffering. There are no limits to the potential outlets for creativity.

Creativity is also a highly effective way of expressing and processing many of the negative feelings generated by chronic pain. Pain can awaken you to start thinking about who you really are and what you are capable of. People claim that the creativity that pain inspires makes them feel better; it strengthens their inner core and frees their true self.

All creative pursuits can support self-discovery, authenticity, and connection with others. Sharing your creative efforts in a group can help you connect and gain a sense of companionship and commonality — social connection is another of the primary pillars that help you cope with chronic pain. Being creative taps directly into your innate potential. It serves to reduce collateral damage and provide positivity, energy, and balance to your losses.

It's important to note that being creative begins with imagining and envisioning creations. If your pain is such that you are quite immobile, then just thinking about some unique creative project can be enough to ease the pain. Your creativity is a fundamental expression of you that can transcend your pain.

Seek the Unchanging Self

Being open to how pain has changed the way you experience yourself creates the possibility of discovering who you are in a deeper sense. Discovering an identity that reflects who you really are despite losses and limitations. Instead of clinging to an old version of yourself that dramatically limits your options, try to open yourself to experience a more authentic version of yourself. There is a human tendency to put our identities into conceptual boxes labeled Job, Religion, Sex, Age, Appearance, or any number of other factors. But the labels reflect only what you are doing in the moment, and each is impermanent. They do not describe the consistent, unchanging thread of who you are.

Your internal growth can be supported by others in your life. Joining with them in this process will have you feeling more connected across the changes in your life, instead of feeling that you've lost yourself and are more disenfranchised. Share your challenges and sense of limitation and frustrations with others. Often you'll find that they can see your qualities and attributes, and your current obstacles to growth, with greater clarity than you can. Process and problem solve with them to help you achieve positive personal change. If you are willing to embrace not knowing who you are for a while, you can push through the limited view of yourself into something larger.

> "Often you'll find that they can see your qualities, attributes, and obstacles with greater clarity than you can."

This growth is rarely pain-free, at least not emotionally so. Observe the amorphous condition of a caterpillar before the butterfly appears! It has an evolutionary-based mechanism for change. Like the butterfly, you too have innate mechanisms for evolution and transformation that can empower you to step outside your comfort zone and explore your potential.

Earlier I shared about Alfred, my client who experienced many losses after his life was interrupted by chronic pain — including the loss of his academic career as a physicist. In the end, few of Alfred's old friends from academia would recognize the man he became. He found a way to teach and write. More importantly, he became less self-centered and more empathic, vulnerable, and compassionate.

Get In On the Remodel

Self-image is a creation developed across your whole life span. It is a work in progress in which you are the architect and general contractor. The onset of chronic pain is not the end of a self-image you can value. A great many of my clients have proven to me that you can choose to deal with the demolition of your old self-image by actively remodeling it. Your new image can be of someone who, despite suffering, has found a way to thrive. This image can be an inspiration to others and a fundamental source of appreciation for yourself. The choice is yours. *The actual damage pain causes to your self-image is a question of choice, not fate.*

Truly Embrace Your Worth

Once you become aware of the truth about the impacts of chronic pain, and dispense with unfounded negative judgments against yourself and other non-user friendly ways of coping, you'll be free to acknowledge that your innate value is based upon having infinite potential. It's not about who you are at any moment in time. Don't brush off compliments on your achievements in recovery as being unjustified or inadequate. They are an expression of your potential. Realize that your efforts in dealing with chronic pain are often heroic. Appreciate your efforts. They are an expression of your sense of purpose and value for life. Applaud yourself! Appreciate your unique qualities. Remind yourself of your essential self every day. Write a list and refer to it often.

> "Realize that your efforts in dealing with chronic pain are often heroic."

If you feel you can't think of anything good about yourself, ask a trusted friend to help you write the list. Remind yourself every day of what you are, and who you strive to be, and that you are worth your struggle to recover.

Concentrate on the value of who you are now. Concentrate on living in the here and now and focusing on possibilities, not limitations. Imagine the future you want, not the one behind you that you can't have. Embrace the work of asserting your needs, wants, feelings, beliefs, and opinions to others in a direct and honest manner. Practice these suggestions every day. It takes effort and vigilance to replace unhelpful thoughts, feelings, and behaviors with healthier versions. Give yourself time to establish new habits. You might keep a diary or journal to chart your progress.

Remove Self-Blame

Shame and guilt are caused by perception. That means you have a great deal of choice about them! Try to appreciate the context in which shame and guilt develop. You and others involved are not the problem.

Recognize that your perceptions of events will trigger feelings and thoughts. These feelings and thoughts may be understandable, but take a hard look at whether their premises might be faulty. Guilt and shame are essentially based on a false premise: that what has happened to you and how you're dealing with it comes with a simple explanation. That it is a failure of your character that is the cause. As this book reveals over and over again, the causes are many and complicated and often not noticed or understood. So are guilt and shame ever really justified?

Consider all the collateral damages that pain has caused you, the often-profound impact it has had on you as a person. Consider all the lack of information or misinformation you have experienced in trying to understand your own dysfunction. *Guilt* and *shame* are words that can imply intentional harm for which you are responsible. But where is your intention to harm, in the reality of the chronic pain experience? There

> "Treat yourself as you would treat your best friend if they were suffering like you are."

is no guilt or shame in not knowing or dealing with something beyond your current ability to cope. Most people with chronic pain just don't realize what they are up against. When they eventually do, their reaction is compassion and empathy for themselves. So treat yourself as you would treat your best friend if they were suffering like you are, as some person deserving of help. Comfort yourself. Be supportive of, kind to, and understanding of yourself!

Enlighten others with knowledge and awareness of the existential truths you've learned about your pain, and then expect the same from them. Ask of yourself and others: *What do I need to help me recover?*

If you think you haven't done enough to recover, ask yourself what typical progress is to be expected in a situation like yours. Most chronic pain sufferers assume they know what's to be expected. And most people tend to trust that their expectations are accurate — even if they're not sure where those expectations came from. But unless you've been through this journey before many times, across many situations, like I and other professionals have, you are likely just making unfounded assumptions.

Feelings of guilt and shame are always based on assumptions, and assumptions are often mistaken. Being hard on yourself because your recovery is slow or stalled is based on an often-false assumption that it's your fault. Challenge your negative self-talk about this. Every time you criticize yourself, stop and look for objective evidence of the accuracy of your criticism.

And don't compare yourself to others. Recognize that, to some extent, every individual's recovery is different.

Rediscover Continuity of Deep Self

Chronic pain doesn't break continuity of self; it changes it. It isn't that you've stopped being you, but that you have lost the sense of yourself as you were. To continue to have a sense of continuity, you must first come to terms and make peace with all the changes your pain has created in who you see yourself to be. This process can be painful and overwhelming at times, but is not at all unsurmountable. Once you have done this, you can rebuild your sense of continuity by becoming aware — through self-exploration — of the aspects of yourself that are not lost by change and challenge unless you choose to let them go: your personal history, your hopes and dreams, your likes, loves, and values, your character, your sense of purpose and inspiration. Self-exploration can be accomplished through different forms of counseling and, more importantly, by engaging in your life in the many ways that reveal you to yourself.

> "Get out of your own way. Don't *struggle* to find out what your purpose is, *explore it.*"

Painful experiences can compel a deeper understanding of your own innate potential to help yourself — your self — heal and recover. Becoming more aware of yourself can reveal a sense of continuity that cannot be changed by circumstances and is always there to help, no matter what the challenge. As a human, you are designed to survive by adapting. Adapt by tapping into your personal power. All the Recovery sections of this book address aspects of this journey. What you need may be skills, but more often is greater awareness of who you are and who you can become.

Be Proactive about Purpose

There are huge rewards in a purpose-driven life. Consider all the concepts associated with purpose: meaning, inspiration, motivation, connection, joy, love, freedom, expanded focus, health, well-being, living in the present, commitment, legacy. How amazing could you and your life be, whether fully embracing or even just tapping into rewards such as these! None of these rewards are out of reach, despite your pain. But conscious work is required to reap them. You can't just think your way into finding your life purpose. Instead, you must become like a professional athlete and put your whole self into it. Practice the techniques and skills offered throughout this book, mindfully and progressively.

The more we act, the more we get clear on things. So don't overthink. Stop with the endless questioning — Will this work out? Should I try that? What if I don't like it? What if I don't make money at it? Instead, create new goals, establish steps to achieve them, and go for it. Get out of your own way. Don't *struggle* to find out what your purpose is, *explore* it. Engage in consistent and proactive action. The experience is the reward, and clarity of purpose will emerge as a natural consequence.

Purpose is found within an exploration of your innate potential. Intuition and self-discovery are part of the process to access this. Start by asking yourself, What matters to me? What stirs my passion? What energizes and inspires me? By connecting to your passions, you will gain insight into what brings you the most sense of purpose. Many of us struggle because we believe that there is *one* thing that we are meant to do, and only one way to do it. This belief is terribly limiting. Let go of it and tap into your ability to redefine and reinvent the ways you find passionate purpose. Let go of thinking there is only one way to feel fulfilled.

My hope is that you can embrace the notion that your purpose in life is to live as fully as you can. Instead of resisting the unknown, embrace it and fully engage in what is happening right here and now, where you are. Passion plus daily action equals a purposeful life.

Choose Your Essential Self

You have not lost your chance to be the person you want to be. The solution lies in realizing that the pain doesn't change the essential you. It may challenge your ideas of who you want to be. But even more, it's challenging you to figure out *how* to be who you want to be, despite the impact of your pain.

You may have to remodel your ideas, to reframe or reimagine how you might embody your desired self, but chronic pain can't take away the qualities that make up who you are. Explore and discover how to find yourself. As with other aspects of recovery, exploring and understanding who you are diminishes the power of pain.

Deepen Your Definition of Satisfaction and Pleasure

Aim for existential, rather than external, satisfaction. Life satisfaction is commonly measured by externals such as wealth, status, career, accomplishments, and possessions. While these things are important, it is what comes from within — your sense of well-being, the quality of your relationships, your self-concept, your self-perceived ability to cope with daily life, and the quantity of pleasurable events you can produce — that gives you *existential* satisfaction. By embracing experiences that reflect your personal values and what you hold important, you can have *meaningful* satisfaction, which is experienced as pleasure.

What can you do, despite your pain, that is within reach and meaningful to you? There is always something. For instance, one of my clients found satisfaction and pleasure by engaging in random acts of curiosity, one of her most cherished values, and in doing so reduced her pain. Another client went from playing baseball to coaching it, enabling him to support his cherished value of teamwork.

An awareness of what really matters to you, and a willingness to think expansively about it, will shape your attitude toward your life as a whole. This can make all the difference!

Practice Enjoyment

To restore and maintain the capacity to enjoy life requires a conscious effort to offset pain's damages to your life and to balance — to your fullest potential — the negative with the positive. This requires a level of self-empowerment and an openness to personal change and evolution.

You can accomplish this by letting go of unhelpful patterns of thinking, feeling, and behaving. Develop more trust in yourself and your ability to live more authentically. Nurture creativity. Use your feelings, senses, and intuition to guide you in recovery, helping you lead your life with vision and inspired action. Devoting a section of your journal to documenting your efforts can be very helpful. Acknowledge each well-taken step; note any surprising results. Enjoying life is a mindset — the result of reflection, action, and gratitude.

Of course, prevention is always more effective than intervention afterward. So, try to adapt to the changes brought by chronic pain as quickly as you can. Develop your capacities for enjoyment. Stimulate and challenge yourself. Make practical, everyday changes. Appreciate the people in your life. Make space to do the things you're best at. The many small changes in your life will soon add up to greater enjoyment.

Chapter 15

Operating-System Impacts

We all have a psychological and emotional "operating system." I liken this to a computer's operating system: In a computer, the operating system is designed to get certain tasks done efficiently and in a user-friendly way. To do this, it uses programs built into the software and hardware. In humans, our system is programmed by organic evolution to help us get all our needs met. The elements of *our* operating system are composed of psychological and emotional operations that support our ability to protect ourselves by positively utilizing our feelings, thoughts, and cognitive abilities.

Chronic pain often does substantial damage to these operations. However, as part of our operating system, we also develop psychological mechanisms that help us to stabilize and cope. Among the most common and useful of these mechanisms are intelligence, practicality, analysis, common sense, organization, resourcefulness, creativity, activity, time management, sensitivity, humor, patience, fortitude, stamina, confidence, focus, discipline, nonjudgmental thinking, and spirituality.

These psychological strategies and skills are necessary for managing the anxiety, anger, and aggression that may arise when unacceptable or potentially harmful experiences and events threaten our needs. Your defense mechanisms are part of your coping system and serve to protect your mind and feelings from damage, as well as your sense of self and your ego. These mechanisms can also provide refuge from situations where you think you can't cope effectively.

This chapter documents specific psychological and emotional impacts caused by chronic pain, impacts that are not in any formal medical or psychological diagnostic category but nonetheless affect your ability to operate effectively as a person. (The more formal and clinical diagnostic categories, like depression, post-traumatic stress disorder, panic attacks, anxiety and anger disorders, and stress will be discussed in chapter 16.)

Though there is some overlap with the emotional and psychological impacts covered in previous chapters, the information provided in this chapter is meant to address more specifically what we usually bring to bear in addressing threats to our needs. The approach to this discussion will refer to the elements of your operating system as they are commonly known — defense mechanisms and coping styles. It is a subject that can be complicated, confusing, and overwhelming. We will focus on these elements and how they can be significantly negatively impacted by your chronic pain, and what to do to counter this. Take heart! Remember, the more detailed and specific your understanding of the impacts of your pain, the more avenues and opportunities you may find to counter them — and to empower yourself.

EROSION OF PSYCHOLOGICAL DEFENSES

Defense mechanisms and coping styles are related to how we perceive and protect ourselves internally, as well as how we are perceived and behave in relation to others. Chronic pain, at its worst, wars with both internal and external perceptions and threatens psychological stability. It makes it hard to invoke and sustain the coping mechanisms you usually depend on. In addition, any of them may require a lot of physical and emotional energy, or be ill-suited to deal with all the damage chronic pain can cause. Chronic pain — by its sheer volume, intensity, and longevity — can "crash" many typical coping systems. I have worked with many dynamic, strong, highly intelligent, and accomplished individuals who have a full comple-ment of excellent traditional coping and defense mechanisms. Just like everyone else, these exceptionally capable individuals find that their coping systems aren't actually designed to deal over time with the destructive power of chronic pain. You need solutions that lie outside of the typical ways of operating and defending yourself.

Meanwhile, as the effectiveness of your usual way of coping declines, you may be tempted to fall back on less helpful strategies. When usual or common mechanisms fail, you may experience an increase in dependency, passivity, and, eventually, a consciousness of helplessness — something I call "the helplessness machine" or "the art of not managing pain." Let's look at some of these less helpful strategies and alternatives to their use.

Disempowering Defenses

When common coping mechanisms for managing stress fail, people often retreat into, or double down on, psychological defenses that can help in the short term but come with major side effects. These side effects can interfere with recovery in the long term and often make your suffering worse.

As you read the list below, ask yourself how well these mechanisms increase your ability to function despite your pain:

Denial is a psychological defense mechanism that avoids confrontation with a personal problem or reality by denying its existence. In other words, a refusal to accept the truth of a reality or experience. The rallying cry of someone in denial is "I can't believe this has happened to me!" Denial prevents you from incorporating unpleasant and unacceptable information about how much you and your life have been damaged by your pain. Denial also stops you from taking these impacts on in a constructive, recovery-oriented fashion. Understandably, you may want to pretend that your life hasn't been altered by pain. But if you live by this pretense, you will be locked down in frustration and unable to change in ways that can lead to new strengths and salvage as much as possible of what has been lost. Acknowledging negative realities is the first step toward empowerment. If you can face the realities in front of you, you can often neutralize, minimize, or even eliminate the impacts. If you deny reality, you will be less likely to look for solutions.

Repression is an attempt to cope by unconsciously forgetting negative information, thoughts, or emotions. Chronic pain threatens many needs. This naturally causes a lot of anxiety, anger, sadness, and negative thoughts. If you automatically block awareness of information, thoughts, and feelings, you lose the chance to use them to help you recover from your pain. Remember, information, thoughts, and feelings are tools in your operating system — they're meant to be used to optimize functioning. They are the lifeblood of coping and recovery.

Suppression is an attempt to ignore information, thoughts, and emotions — especially anxiety, anger, sadness, loss, and stress — by putting them out of your awareness. You may not want to acknowledge how you feel or what has happened to you. That's understandable. You may think expressing negative thoughts or emotions is a weakness, or that somehow it would be "giving in" to the pain. However, you will find that allowing yourself to embrace your emotional pain, as you would if you were grieving, can free you to move on and recover. In truth, it is essential that you own what has happened to you and how you've been affected emotionally, and that you put it out there for yourself and others to know. This is one of the major steps toward personal empowerment.

Intellectualization is neutralizing your feelings of anxiety, anger, or sadness by "thinking away" these emotions or any other reaction you don't want to feel. This coping mechanism includes rationalizing or adopting ideas that minimize how you are being affected emotionally. This is quite different from engaging in analysis of problems, synthesis of information, and problem-solving and creative solutions, in which emotions are the fuel that drives these cognitive processes. This alignment can help you tap into your true potential to help yourself recover.

Avoidance is a coping mechanism characterized by the effort to escape thinking about or dealing with information, thoughts, and feelings. With chronic pain, you can only avoid what has happened and is happening to you for so long. Eventually, it will catch up with you. The time lost in putting off dealing with chronic pain will only make things worse: Managing chronic pain requires absolute engagement — not avoidance. When you engage the impacts, you can bring to bear all your psychological and emotional resources to help yourself.

Withdrawal/hiding means distancing yourself from fear and other emotions by way of a psychological and sometimes physical separation from situations or other people. By withdrawing, you save yourself from having to communicate with others. But this situation works against your needs and self-interest. You pay for the sought-for "safety" with loneliness and alienation. Your best hope is to turn and face things, fully connected to yourself and all others involved in your pain problem. Emotional connection and support from others is one of the most important elements of successful recovery.

Distraction is diverting attention away from a stressor and toward other unrelated thoughts or behaviors. While distraction may be temporarily helpful, overuse of distraction leads away from, not toward, long-lasting solutions. And chronic pain eats away at distraction like acid on metal. There's an expiration date on how often and how much you can distract yourself. Paying attention to the impacts of chronic pain may be physically and emotionally uncomfortable and stressful, but it can also inspire you to seek more information from your providers and to engage in proactive, recovery-oriented activities that can lessen your impacts and reduce your pain.

Inactivity is the absence of action, the lack of will to act, or the adoption of a passive approach to a problem. Inactivity will just add to your losses and make it harder to recover. Dealing with chronic pain requires action and major activity — both physical and emotional.

Impulsivity is acting out your desires or other feelings, especially extreme anger or anxiety, with little regard for consequences. This approach often compounds the stress of chronic pain and limits access to your higher cognitive and emotional faculties, which could otherwise help you recover. While it's understandable when your fears and suffering motivate you to act out, being intentional and following a plan is more likely to bring relief and recovery.

Regression is reverting to a childlike state of development or dependency, and childlike behaviors, under conditions of stress. The road rage you see when drivers are stuck in traffic is like a child having a temper tantrum; it's a great example of regression. Assuming a stance toward others like that of a dependent or helpless child — for example, wholly delegating to others your personal responsibility for dealing with your challenges — is another example of regression. This outcome can be encouraged and compounded when others' actions are disempowering and infantilizing. It's actually common for people to interpret a person in pain as some kind of dependent (the "child") being taken care of by their providers (the "adults" in the room). In reality, you, your supportive others, and your providers are teammates, and you will serve your recovery better by being an adult and "co-parenting" with them.

Dissociation is a defense mechanism in which you momentarily lose connection to the world around you. You feel separated from the outside world and other people, and cope with uncomfortable situations by psychologically removing yourself from them. Chronic pain can be traumatic, which can push you toward dissociation, but disconnection means disempowerment. Instead, focus on processing the emotional impact of your pain, and you'll make it unnecessary to use this defense.

Psychological isolation is a defense mechanism that separates certain awareness, knowledge, and ideas or feelings from the rest of your thoughts. The typical experience of someone with chronic pain, as outlined throughout this book, often evokes this defense, often by default rather than by desire. You may find it temporarily helpful to use rationalizations, assumptions, or downright magical thinking to try to protect yourself against future suffering. For example, you endorse negative pain beliefs like "I'll always be in pain!" or "I'm helpless!" You create negative belief systems ("No matter what I do, it's not good enough!") and also negative judgments ("I'm weak and lazy!"). These thoughts may seem logical and legitimate and absolve you of personal responsibility for your recovery. Unfortunately, they are also disempowering and de-motivating. They narrow your range of recovery options and constructive actions. Don't forget, *you* get to decide how you want to think about your pain and its impacts. If you seek to be authentic, accurate, and truthful in your thoughts, they can help you to be less stressed and more empowered to recover.

Social isolation pursues coping by limiting contact with others. The only thing worse than having chronic pain is having to live with it all by yourself. Emotional support is one of the most critical ways of being able to thrive with chronic pain. Dealing with chronic pain, just like any other natural disaster, does take a village.

Sleep, as a method of relief from your pain and suffering and an escape from an unbearable wakefulness, is understandable as a coping mechanism. However, when sleep is not strictly restorative, it becomes a real impediment to the time, energy, and commitment you need to put into your recovery. Sleep may also become less restful if pain and worries cause fitfulness or unpleasant dreams that wake you and become emotionally draining.

Passivity is inaction, mental or physical, in the face of suffering. When you engage in passivity, you become the object of experience rather than the actor. For example, you may become inactive, isolate yourself socially, and withdraw from others. Passivity is also seen in relying on forms of treatment that are received passively. Using pharmaceuticals or relaxation massage, chiropractic or acupuncture, can be a form of passivity if not combined with more active treatment such as physical reconditioning or counseling. Though it may be hard to believe, you have the power, in many ways, to determine whether chronic pain defeats you, or whether you master your pain and gain a continued life of thriving. To do this, you must be extremely active in your participation in recovery.

Safety behaviors are behaviors used to reduce anxiety and fear by escaping potentially uncomfortable physical or emotional situations. For example, putting off treatment, engaging in excessive downtime, procrastinating, or practicing guarding and protecting behaviors (like grimacing, moving with exaggerated care, grasping or clutching for physical support and safety, moaning or calling out, and flinching when being touched). These behaviors are maladaptive over the long term because they prolong anxiety and may produce negative side effects. For example, you may think, "I know there's something wrong with me physically, but I'm afraid to go to the doctor." Putting it off helps in the moment — but then you begin to worry: "What if there is really something wrong with me, and I'm delaying treatment?" Delaying treatment can magnify the problem.

Wishing is expressing a strong desire or hope for something that may not be attainable, or something that cannot or probably will not happen without action being taken. Recovery requires a high level of personal action and effort to produce the desired outcomes. You have the capability to take this on. You are not a beggar, and wishes are not horses you can ride to recovery.

Bargaining is an attempt to negotiate the pain or illness away by being willing to do *anything* not to feel it anymore. This can lead to doctor-shopping, either using multiple doctors to get drugs or switching from one doctor to another to avoid an unwanted opinion. (Doctor-shopping doesn't mean carefully searching to find an appropriate match.) Bargaining can also lead to drug abuse, experimental procedures, and investment in unrealistic promises or expectations, and other actions that only delay or counter any action toward recovery.

Pleading is where you beg, to someone or some belief, for life to be what it once was. It's being willing to offer anything to make your illness or pain go away or give you some semblance of the life you once had. Pleading might sound something like *"Please just don't let this ruin my life"* or *"If you make the pain go away, I promise I'll be a better person."* This type of thinking is ultimately disempowering.

Depression as a defense mechanism is a complex means for suppressing anxiety and anger. Depression is a state where emotions eventually shut down, reducing access to critically important emotions that you will need for your recovery. Allowing clinical (debilitating, long-lasting) depression to continue untreated invites a whole host of symptoms that further undermine functioning.

Despair is the complete loss or absence of hope — disheartenment, desperation, misery, defeatism, pessimism. Sometimes despair is rooted in the idea that you are helpless, a perception that is never accurate. Why? It is contrary to our biological programming and our will to survive, and it's self-defeating. There are always options; they just may not be ones that you like. But starting somewhere is better than being unwilling to move, in any way, toward recovery.

Substance abuse is the excessive use of recreational drugs, alcohol, cigarettes, comfort foods, or other emotional crutches to alleviate symptoms of mental distress, stress, and anxiety. The goal is to make you forget the reality of what's happening in your life. These coping methods create more side effects than they alleviate, and they will undermine your life functioning well beyond any difficulties caused by your pain.

Enabling behaviors are dysfunctional behaviors that are intended to help resolve a specific problem but in fact may perpetuate or exacerbate the problem. They may take the form of not taking responsibility, or of making unjustified rationalizations for disempowering conduct. Some common enabling behaviors among people living with chronic pain are engaging in substance abuse, letting others help them without trying themselves, or even feigning helplessness and trying to guilt others into helping. Enabling behaviors aim to deny the harm your choices may create. They also block access to the internal need or pressure to change. Other people, from family members to providers, can also engage in enabling behaviors, including solicitous thoughts and emotional or physical behaviors that — no matter how well intentioned — justify or reinforce your limited functioning and disability. These behaviors include not being honest about their own feelings, needs, or perspective to "protect" the person with pain from feeling bad about their limitations, treating the person with pain as if they're disabled, and even preempting the person with pain from being more active out of fear or misunderstanding of the person's true ability to function.

Counterproductive Coping Styles

In addition to our list of defense mechanisms, we all have a preferred coping style — encompassing personality traits, beliefs, and orientations — that can either help or hinder recovery. Below is a sampling of style components most likely to work against someone trying to recover from chronic pain, and alternatives to them. As you read, consider to what extent these components are a part of your personal style:

Stoicism is the control of negative emotions by being unemotional or acting indifferent, enduring without complaint, or "being tough" beyond the point that it is helpful. The idea of pushing through the obstacles in your chronic pain by sheer force of will and determination can be a powerful personality trait in certain situations. It's also limited — in both application and durability — and often poorly suited to the situation. Stoicism also requires a tremendous amount of personal energy, especially when combating major stressors. In chronic pain, stoicism often distracts from real solutions, especially ones that require personal growth. Personal evolution is the key to successful recovery, and stoicism can be an obstacle to this. The alternative to a misuse of stoicism is being open to your challenges and working to reduce them, not just bear them.

Passive aggression is characterized by expressing negative feelings of anger and anxiety in an indirect, unassertive, or concealed way. Sarcasm, procrastination, and stubbornness are forms of passive aggression when used to prevent yourself or others from knowing how you really feel and what you really need. But remember: The expression of both feelings and needs is essential to recovery. Being angry is understandable, considering the damage pain does to your life. To show respect for these feelings, express them in a manner that can lead to resolution — not confusion.

Aggression covers a range of destructive behaviors that can result in both physical and psychological harm to yourself, others, or objects in your environment. For instance, using anger to keep yourself and others at arm's length, or directing anger at yourself and rejecting or criticizing offered help to prevent others (and yourself) from seeing your fear and vulnerability. In addition, aggressive behavior distracts from your awareness of your own needs and reduces access to needed support. Because chronic pain threatens so many needs, it's easy to succumb to this way of channeling your feelings. But aggression is destructive. It will cause you to lose touch with those aspects of yourself that can help. If you focus your anger constructively toward reconstruction instead of demolition, it will help reduce the threats to your needs and ground you in your full potential to deal with your pain.

Hysteria is a word used to describe a range of shallow, volatile emotions and overdramatic or attention-seeking behaviors. It is a word both historically and currently overassigned to women, but the concept remains useful for describing a type of behavior that can be engaged in by anyone of any gender. Catastrophic thinking, which distorts and amplifies negative emotions, threats, and the actual pain experience, is a type of hysteria. Hysteria undermines your ability to participate in treatment and benefit from it. It may alienate the very people you need help from by leading them to think of you as less accurate and therefore less believable about your actual experience. Hysteria may also lead to experiencing increased anxiety and self-doubt. The sky is only falling if you decide it is. You get to decide how to experience what is happening to you and how to talk about it. You can avoid hysteria if you practice the many techniques described in this book to calm and center yourself, such as techniques for meditation, accurate thinking, and constructively addressing your anxiety.

Alienation is the perception or reality of being misunderstood, rejected, separate from, or marginalized by other individuals or some larger segment of society. This can refer to psychological or emotional separation as well as physical separation. People with chronic pain often feel alone and isolated in their experience, and this substantially amplifies their suffering. As I've said, and will say again, this stance is a choice — not an inevitability. Alienation breeds resentment and a tendency to move away from others, along with a lack of willingness to really engage in difficult treatments and demanding personal changes. There are many ways to communicate your physical pain and emotional suffering — and to experience empathy from others, which is the remedy for alienation. Remember that everyone has experienced some physical pain and emotional suffering. It's what unites us as humans.

Counter-dependencies are behaviors and thoughts that convey a refusal of attachment, or the denial of personal needs and dependency. For example, acting like you don't need anyone. Chronic pain recovery cannot be handled alone. Acting like you're okay and trying to handle it all yourself will inevitably lead to difficulty. It's not shameful or weak to know that you need help, to ask for it, and to accept it.

Perfectionism is a negative belief that people will think less of you if you make a mistake. That you are less worthwhile if you fail. You believe people will look down on you if they find out about all the mistakes you've made. You get upset if you make a mistake and feel you should be perfect. Recovery requires you to appreciate the imperfect nature of being human and to see your "flaws" as an invitation to evolve. The belief system that is perfectionism prevents that. Remember that chronic pain is about damage control. Let your imperfection guide you to recovery-based personal growth.

Self-criticism and self-blame are negative belief structures that make you feel guilty if someone is annoyed with you. You criticize yourself for not getting along well with a friend or family member. You blame yourself for problems in relationships. If someone's upset with you, you feel like it's your fault. Chronic pain causes dysfunction in relationships — that's a fact. You need to be able to address this objectively and without assuming fault or guilt. This will allow you to work through the challenges chronic pain presents and to maintain your relationships. In fact, there's a real opportunity to deepen relationships by working through the challenges chronic pain presents in terms of how you think about yourself. This growth can happen only in the absence of self-criticism and self-blame. You can start by learning the rules for conflict resolution.

Entitlement is a negative belief that you deserve better treatment from others. You may get upset when people do not fulfill your expectations. You may believe others are to blame for the problems in your relationships with them. Perhaps you often get frustrated or annoyed with people. In chronic pain, this belief can be particularly problematic in your efforts to get your needs met with providers, friends, and family, who are often unsure of how to help or feel limited in their power to help you. Expecting to be treated well in the treatment environment — without effort on your part — is a risky proposition. Expecting others to treat you as if you're special, expecting them to know what you're dealing with and what you need, will doom you to disappointment! If you know how to positively address your disappointments with others — for example, through conflict resolution techniques — you can avoid falling into this situation.

Approval addiction is a negative belief that your self-esteem depends more on what others think of you than on what you think. It leads to criticism and disapproval from others being excessively upsetting and you feeling worthless and defensive. Chronic pain undermines many aspects of functioning, and if you base your self-esteem on others' approval, it is likely to erode. However, you are the best judge of your worth. No limitation should be used to disqualify you. Your power to recover depends on the degree to which you can unconditionally love yourself.

Love addiction is a negative belief that you cannot feel happy or fulfilled without being loved by another person. You believe that if you're not loved, you're bound to be unhappy. If someone rejects you, there must be something wrong with you. You must be loved to be a worthwhile human being, and being alone is bound to lead to unhappiness. Thus, when chronic pain disables much of your ability to please others, you may believe you cannot satisfy your need for love. However, loving yourself, by definition, is not conditioned on anything other than your existence.

Low self-esteem is a negative belief that you will never feel truly happy or worthwhile. If you're one who holds this belief, then chronic pain will feed it, and it will disempower you. Remember, chronic pain challenges you existentially. It demands that you decide who you really are. If you are inclined to lower your self-worth based on what you can or cannot do, take every chance to reverse that thinking. Acknowledge something you value in yourself instead.

Achievement addiction is a negative belief that people who achieve a great deal are more worthwhile than those who do not. You may feel inferior to people who are more intelligent and successful than you are. Perhaps your self-esteem depends greatly on how productive and successful you are compared to others. Given the obstacles to achievement that chronic pain creates, this belief will significantly compound your stress. Try to remove the component of achievement from your self-worth. Instead, consider achievement a preference. Let your desire to achieve be based on your will to live and thrive.

Helplessness and hopelessness are negative beliefs in which you feel pessimistic that things could ever change for the better. Perhaps you believe it will be extremely difficult or impossible to solve the problems in your life. You believe that your bad moods result from factors beyond your control, and that there's little anyone can do to help you solve your problems. This set of beliefs is anathema to recovery and absolutely works against you. You are never helpless, and you cannot be hopeless unless you've completely run out of imagination.

Negative judgmental self-talk is self-defeating internal chatter that combines conscious thoughts with unconscious beliefs and biases. It is a typical reaction, in our society, to the limitations and suffering that chronic pain brings. However, judgmental self-talk muddies the psychological waters and dilutes your natural abilities to find solutions. It is essential that you discover the truth in your experience instead.

Emotional guardedness is a habit of guarding against vulnerability by keeping a tight rein on expressing your feelings, thoughts, or dreams, or in any way exposing the real you. To recover, it's essential that you be open to yourself and others about how you feel about your condition and what you need. Vulnerability is the common human denominator. We are all, at all times, vulnerable to all kinds of threats. Vulnerability—when expressed authentically—is something everyone understands and should respect, and it's not a mark of weakness. Feigning invulnerability is to pretend you're not human. Making peace with your own vulnerability can be a powerfully positive thing, and can level the playing field with everyone involved in helping and caring about you.

Lack of awareness is a reduced consciousness of one's own body and state of mind, including one's thoughts, actions, ideas, feelings, and interactions with others. Behaviors that reveal a lack of awareness include:

- Inattention to extreme emotions, thoughts, and behaviors
- Lack of awareness of emotional balance
- Limited knowledge of emotional control and impact of thoughts
- Limited awareness of the function of emotions
- Avoidance or aggression when dealing with negative emotions
- Impulsive expressions of emotion and behaviors
- Emotional interruptions of attention and focus

Lack of awareness contributes to limited possibilities and emotional instability that perpetuate limits to optimal operating as a person. Awareness is necessary to promoting emotional, psychological, and physical recovery. It allows you to measure your needs, progress, and risks. It encourages creativity and innovation. To begin to move into awareness is both a physical, intellectual, and emotional experience. Exercise, meditate, explore, ask questions. Pay attention to what is happening to you, others, and your world. A heightened level of awareness in all of this will produce more helpful decisions and actions.

UNRESOLVED CHILDHOOD PATTERNS

My clients are often confused as to why their personal history and development are part of their initial evaluation. Chronic pain is often experienced as a dependent state reminiscent of childhood, where you're dependent upon "adults" to help get you out of your suffering. The behavior of your medical caregivers, family, and friends, no matter how well intended, may remind you of negative experiences with caregivers as you were growing up. If this happens, your pain may resonate with and resurface old emotional wounds and unresolved issues. It may evoke earlier developed dysfunctional patterns of coping. In this way, stress from the past is added to your present pain.

Unwittingly, you may experience and repeat familiar patterns that evoke anxiety, frustration, and resistance to recommended treatment plans and help from others. Your past matters! Without understanding how it may contribute to your current pain and ability to cope, it can revive and reactivate past traumatic events and behaviors, which now become associated with your current pain, exacerbating it and confounding treatment without anyone knowing or understanding its potential for negative impact. This cycle often goes unexplored and unaddressed.

In this situation, it's often the case that no one has a clue as to what's really happening—not even you.

For example, suppose you never got to feel truly taken care of as a child. Now chronic pain creates a need to be dependent on others, and you may unconsciously seek to perpetuate those circumstances, by taking a helpless, passive approach to managing your pain, slowing down your own recovery without knowing it. Or there may be self-esteem or identity issues, attachment issues, or dysfunctional patterns of conflict and emotional management that resonate with your painful circumstances now. A history of traumatic experiences in childhood, especially sexual, physical, and emotional abuse, can interfere with treatment success. This is especially the case when providers ask patients to endure pain and suffering during treatment "for their own good."

Resurfacing of the past is often misunderstood or even ignored by providers and patients alike, all while old and unresolved emotional issues add to the traumatic and complicated nature of managing your pain.

EMOTIONAL DYSREGULATION

The multiple threats to your needs caused by chronic pain, even in the most well-balanced person, can cause destabilization of your successful utilization of emotions. This can cause a major disruption to your ability to operate effectively, through a loss of consistent management and regulation of an important part of your operating system. Over time, chronic pain's longevity erodes your emotional scaffolding. This change is often hard to recognize, unexpected, and poorly understood. It may come about from the sheer number of threats to your needs from your pain as well as arise from your individual history.

Negative experiences with caregivers in formative years can establish patterns conducive to emotional dysregulation in adult life. Emotional dysregulation can also be triggered by negative reactions to your condition from friends, caregivers, and co-workers. For example, if a caregiver interacts in a way that is overprotective, controlling, critical, solicitous, or unpredictable.

Another factor that contributes to emotional dysregulation is holding any of a number of common but disempowering pain beliefs, which will be explained below.

Emotional dysregulation can cause emotional volatility, from relatively minor to extreme. Here are some examples:

- Difficulty calming yourself down when upset
- Experiencing more negative emotions and focusing on them
- Difficulty decreasing your negative emotions
- Becoming avoidant or aggressive when dealing with negative emotions
- Impulsive, emotional interruption of attention and focus
- Difficulty managing emotional experience

NEGATIVE BELIEFS AND NEGATIVE SELF-TALK

Negative beliefs both about pain and about yourself often multiply when you are experiencing chronic pain. They are the product of who you are, your personal history, your belief systems, and how you perceive your experience of pain, and interaction with providers, treatment, and the interpersonal environment.

However, negative beliefs disempower you and drain you emotionally. They obscure the truth in many situations, and color your perception of self and others. Negative beliefs are not a true reflection of your character. They are an emotional reaction to your negative experiences with pain, treatment, and recovery, filtered through who you are and how you think.

The following is a list of typical negative pain beliefs that may develop in relation to your pain, your reaction to it, your interaction with treatment, and the reaction of others in your life:

- I will always be in pain.
- I am back to square one again. Nothing I do makes a difference (or will make a difference, or has made a difference). Things just keep getting worse.

- I can't function like this.
- It's no use trying anymore.
- It's too hard to stay in shape to prevent pain flare-ups, too hard to do the exercises, too inconvenient to stay with the program.
- The pain is intolerable. I can't stand it.
- I'm being punished.
- It's all my fault.
- I don't deserve this.
- This pain I just felt means I'm going to have a bad flare-up.
- This pain I just felt means I've done something terrible to my body.
- I'm weak.
- I'm going to be disabled.
- The problems causing my pain are too complex for anyone to understand.
- Nothing ever changes.
- Nobody cares.
- This is just not fair. It shouldn't be this way.
- They (those people over there) deserve to be in pain. I don't!
- I can't handle this. I can't cope.
- I'll never be able to go back to work. My life will be ruined.
- I may have overdone it. I need to quit. I need to lie in bed.
- Why should I have to work so hard at not being in pain? No one else I know has to.

In general, your beliefs about your pain alter your perception of it. Those beliefs have a strong effect on how much pain you feel, and on how much your pain sabotages your ability to function.

Please understand this: There is a proven correlation. Beliefs can make you fearful of the pain itself, fearful of activity and its effect on pain, and fearful of reinjuring yourself. Your beliefs can make you afraid of rehabilitation — and afraid for your life. Beliefs and perceptions can convince you that you're disabled and leave you feeling helpless, hopeless, and possessed by your pain.

In addition to negative beliefs, you may develop negative self-talk about yourself and others. Going about our daily lives, we're constantly thinking about and interpreting the situations we find ourselves in and how we perceive ourselves and others. It's as though we have an internal voice inside our head that determines how we perceive every situation. Psychologists call this inner voice "self-talk," and it includes our conscious thoughts as well as our unconscious assumptions or beliefs.

Much of our self-talk is reasonable: "I'd better do some preparation for that exam," or "I'm really looking forward to that match." However, some of it is negative, unrealistic, or self-defeating: "I'm going to fail for sure," or "I didn't play well! I'm hopeless." Name-calling — calling yourself a failure, a loser, stupid, a jerk, negligent, lazy, a procrastinator, or weak — is the worst form of negative self-talk.

Overall, our self-talk is often skewed toward the negative, and it is largely just plain inaccurate. So it's extremely useful to keep an eye on how you think about your experience. Be prepared to challenge some of the inaccurate negative aspects of your thinking. If you notice yourself magnifying the negative aspects of a situation and filtering out all the positive aspects, try to catch yourself and correct that. If something unpleasant or disappointing occurs, do you automatically blame yourself? When you hear that an evening out with friends is canceled, do you assume that the change in plans is because no one wanted to be around you?

In chronic pain, the tendency toward all-or-nothing thinking is like an epidemic that sickens us. With this kind of thinking we automatically anticipate the worst about ourselves and/or others, and see things only as good or bad, people only as heroes or villains, perfect or a failure. We lose our sense of a middle ground.

RECOVERY: HEALTHY MANAGEMENT OF OPERATING SYSTEMS

Chronic pain is a call to action, innovation, and personal evolution. If you narrowly conceptualize chronic pain as a purely physical phenomenon (instead of something that also affects the non-physical and cumulatively traumatic aspects of your life), you will likely underestimate what you're up against. This makes you susceptible to ineffective ideas, nonproductive psychological and emotional reactions, and behavior that can work against your recovery. But remember: To deal with existential threats, you need existential defenses. You need a new strategy for using your common defenses, or alternative approaches that can increase your psychological and physical functioning while boosting your emotional strength. Here are five steps toward recovery.

Choose Your Defenses and Refine Your Personal Style

This list of time-tested, core concepts is central to all approaches proven to work effectively in the management of chronic pain:

- Acknowledge the negative realities of your situation.
- Cultivate the ability to be completely truthful with yourself.

- Be true to who you are (authenticity).
- Practice constructive emotional management.
- Find comfort with vulnerability.
- Cultivate positive dependence upon others.
- Proactively seek help and support.
- Value your innate self unconditionally.
- Value effort and intention over achievement.
- Have a sense of purpose and inspiration.

As we've come to understand, chronic pain is like a tsunami, an earthquake, or a 9/11 event. Because its impacts are multiple and severe, extraordinary measures must be taken to deal with them. For psychological and emotional recovery, you need to be able to utilize all the psychological defense mechanisms, personal styles, traits, beliefs, and orientations that work in support of recovery. These strategies are the core of managing chronic pain successfully. They often require self-reflection, self-development, and the evolution of your current operating system.

Protect Cognition

There are many techniques and approaches that can be used to address cognitive dysfunction caused by your pain, all of which are thoroughly covered in chapter 8. Be sure to make protecting your cognitive processes an integral part of your plan. These processes are part of your operating system, and at the core of your ability to use your thoughts, knowledge, wisdom, and awareness in aid of mastering your pain.

Put Old Issues to New Use

Unintegrated traumatic experiences or negative associations from childhood will affect your ability to trust and depend on others, and to effectively cope in the present. If these issues have not been resolved, they will resurface and add to the difficulty of managing your pain in the present. I have seen hundreds of cases where this has occurred. When past issues — unknown to providers — cause treatment to fail, providers may label patients as "treatment resistant," "courting secondary gain," or just plain "malingering." Even worse, their patients may end up thinking they are responsible for the failure of their treatment.

Counseling is often required to expose, process, and work through your unhealed issues. Otherwise, these issues, operating outside your awareness — and your providers' awareness — will cause misunderstandings. They will confuse your perception of yourself, your pain, your reactions to pain, and your understanding of others. It's essential to analyze these unique elements of your personal history in order to assess how they may contribute to your experience of pain, and whether they might undermine treatment and recovery.

I will also say this: There are many added benefits of counseling for these issues, including the strengthening of your identity, personal integration, confidence, and your ability to cope.

Build the Skill of Emotional Regulation

Emotional regulation depends on several things:

- Being able to acknowledge what's happened to you
- Knowing how to manage your negative emotional reactions when your needs are threatened
- Being compassionate with yourself

To build these skills, engage in self discovery and the evolution of your operating system. Seek empowering environments — ideally, places and people that offer opportunities to practice without overstimulation or excessive frustration. Your goal is to better understand yourself and your needs and how to get them met. You need to be comfortable with being open and unashamed about your feelings, and in asking for what you need and telling others what can be helpful to you. This will aid you in reclaiming your ability to maintain emotional regulation.

Effective strategies to help you do this are to practice being aware of your feelings, moment by moment, to acknowledge all your challenges and any opportunities to address them, and to work at being empathic toward others. For those around you who want to help in this, trying to model this level of awareness with authentic involvement is more likely to inspire you. Everyone involved can make an effort to respect the difficulties of maintaining emotional equilibrium during the existential challenges of chronic pain.

Deliberately Counter Negativity

Negative emotions, especially anxiety and anger, happen in reaction to the damage to your needs that pain creates. The negative emotions alert you to this damage, which means if you use them properly, you can help reduce damage. Emotions are there to help you become more aware of the accuracy of your thoughts and to help you take the optimal actions to deal with them.

However, negative *beliefs* drain your emotional, psychological, and physical energy. They are almost always a distortion of reality. They pollute your consciousness. They sap your motivation and ability to act proactively and constructively toward the challenges you face. If these beliefs are based on your negative experiences in treatment, you can learn to take a more empowered, proactive approach in treatment situations. (For more on interacting in the treatment environment, see chapters 17 and 18.)

Dealing with negative beliefs often requires the help of a counselor. Together, you can explore the origin of the belief systems that generate negative thoughts, then work to eliminate them from your operating system. This work often involves cognitive coping techniques, which are also often offered in pain-management counseling. With these techniques, you will be able to replace inaccurate negative thoughts with objective, rational, unbiased truth. This will be extremely helpful in your recovery. As you become a true partner to your providers in treatment, you can dispel many of the illusions that pain creates. With your providers, you can test, challenge, and change your pain beliefs.

> "You'll probably be surprised by how much of your thinking reflects only the negatives of your situation and none of the positives."

Here are a few practices to get started: Beware of assumptions. Notice the premise upon which your negative self-talk is based as it happens. Ask yourself if your negative beliefs and self-talk reflect the true reality of the situation and the objective, verified facts.

Learning to dispute assumptions and negative thoughts takes time and practice. But it's worth the effort. Doing so aligns your stress with your actual experience, and usually reduces your stress and increases your ability to cope. Once you start examining your assumptions, you'll probably be surprised by how much of your thinking reflects only the negatives of your situation and none of the positives, and is filled with inaccuracies and exaggerations.

Use your good intellect. Challenge your runaway mind and the feelings it creates. Use your feelings as a guide to the accuracy and clarity of your perceptions. Ground and center yourself with questions that help you figure out whether your self-talk is reasonable and if the premises for your feelings are based on reality. This will give you greater authority and control with which to confront and overcome your challenges. Understanding exactly what you're up against is half the solution to a problem. Using the tools provided by your innate potential in an optimal way is the other half. Who and what you are and what you know will address the problems at whatever level they manifest.

Here are four main strategies for self-questioning:

(1) **Test reality:**

- What is my evidence for and against my thinking?
- What facts are my thoughts based on?
- How am I interpreting the situation? Could there be other interpretations?
- Am I jumping to negative conclusions?
- How can I find out if my thoughts are true?

(2) **Look for alternative explanations:**

- What other ways can I look at this situation?
- What else could this mean?
- If I were being positive, how would I perceive this situation?

(3) **Put things in perspective:**

- Is this situation as bad as I'm making it out to be?
- What is the worst thing that could happen? How likely is it?
- What's the best thing that could happen?
- What is most likely to happen?
- Is there anything good about this situation?
- How will this make a difference in five years' time?

When you feel anxious, depressed, or stressed out, your self-talk is likely to become even more extreme. You'll be more likely to expect the worst and focus on the most negative aspects of your situation. So it's helpful to try and put things into their proper perspective.

(4) **Use goal-directed thinking:**

- How is thinking this way helping me to feel good or to achieve my goals?
- What can I do that will help me solve the problem?
- Is there something I can learn from this situation to help me do it better next time?

Recognize that your current way of thinking might be self-defeating — it doesn't make you feel good or help you get what you want. This realization can sometimes motivate you to look at things from a different perspective. You are the master of what you think and how you perceive your experience.

Chapter 16

Mental Health Impacts and Risk Factors

It will be no surprise to most people with chronic pain to hear that persistent, unresolved pain can cause mental health problems. This includes mood, anxiety, and anger disorders as well as depression, panic attacks, and PTSD. If you are experiencing any of these, they can also dramatically add to your pain. They undermine treatment, inhibit recovery, and decrease your ability to function.

This chapter will discuss childhood risk factors for mental health, then outline some of the most prevalent mental health impacts from chronic pain, how they manifest, and various ways to prevent them from occurring or to recover from them. Following the existential approach used throughout this book, I present these impacts as problems with solutions. This means that we look at them as more than just a diagnosis and a list of symptoms. Mental health impacts are events in your life with meaning and purpose. As you proceed, consider how this approach, in addition to the more conventional approaches, can help you. Remember, solutions will be explained in the Recovery section.

MENTAL HEALTH RISK FACTORS

Risk factors are events and experiences in childhood and other developmental years that can make it more likely for someone's pain experience and treatment outcomes to be more negative and/or more prolonged. As will be explained, risk factors involve aspects of your history that can affect how you perceive pain, how much pain you experience, how you respond to treatment, and how well you will be able to cope with it. They are all part of experiences that can create a destabilizing effect on your mastery of pain and make it more likely you will fall victim to it. Each of them can be addressed and resolved, but it is important to note that they have all been found to be a part of the equation for understanding the different ways that chronic pain affects people.

As I have said many times before, who you are as a unique individual is of critical importance in understanding and helping you with your pain. Who you are includes your personal history: experiences in childhood, your teen years, and some adult years that can significantly influence how you perceive your pain and communicate and cope with it. This influence is particularly notable in situations where you experience your chronic pain as a newer version of old, unresolved, and unexpressed emotional pain or dysfunctional thinking and behavior. The following are the major risk factors to look out for:

Abandonment. Childhood fears of abandonment (even if unconscious) can be triggered in adulthood by treatment providers or significant others. This can make you anxious about asserting your needs or being vulnerable, or cause fears of being rejected or cast out. These difficult emotions can undermine your recovery.

Divorce. If, during your childhood, your parents had a contentious relationship or divorce, it may have undermined your ability to feel secure about getting your needs met or engaging in the successful resolution of conflicts. These historical issues may get in the way of successfully getting help with your pain. Your early experience may leave you with conflict avoidance or lacking a healthy sense of entitlement concerning your pain-related needs.

Harsh, punitive, distant, cold parents. If you had parental experiences like these, it may have left you with a challenged sense of self-worth and a low expectation of positive treatment from others. This background may also cause difficulties with trust. All of this can make it hard for you to get needed support from others and good care in treatment.

Physical and/or sexual abuse. Early abuse can have a major negative impact on how you experience medical treatment, especially hands-on treatments by someone insensitive to the issue of abuse. This is more likely to arise when the treatment itself causes more physical or emotional pain or when you're told "It's for your own good" or "Learn to live with it." You may end up experiencing the whole treatment environment as abusive — with predictably negative consequences to your recovery.

Neglect. If you felt neglected as a child, this can create self-worth issues and antagonism toward authority figures. These are issues that can seriously complicate you getting what you need from providers and others. It may lead to dysfunctional methods of coping as well.

Trauma. Chronic pain and disappointments in treatment can become traumatic for anyone. If you've suffered earlier trauma, especially unresolved trauma, your current experience can create a resonance in which your pain becomes a channel for old emotional wounds. This will aggravate your present pain.

Early parentification. People who were cast in a parent role at an early age can be left with a need to be super responsible, unselfish, and self-reliant to a fault. This can make it very difficult for you ask for what you need, or to trust and depend on caregivers and supportive others during your chronic pain. It can undermine your own ability to help yourself recover, and possibly produce negative reactions in those whose help you need.

Interpersonal conflict. A childhood experience of excessive amounts of conflict without positive resolution can create negative expectations for managing the inevitable conflicts that arise with others in a chronic pain situation.

Loss. If you suffered significant loss as a child, especially emotionally unprocessed and unresolved loss, that experience could add negative emotional weight to the multiple losses caused by chronic pain and potentially cause greater emotional disability.

Parental substance abuse. If you witnessed substance-abuse behaviors as an ongoing problem during childhood, this can set the stage for dysfunctional coping patterns regarding the use of pain medications and other substances.

Parental or sibling mental health issues. Excessive familial mental health challenges during childhood can contribute to a lack of self-worth, stability, attention, and consistency in adult life. This can negatively impact the development of your ability to cope successfully and get your needs met.

Chronic illness/pain in the family. Chronic illness or pain in childhood, dealt with in dysfunctional ways, may contribute to unsuccessful patterns of managing pain. How your caretakers addressed challenges for themselves — perhaps they behaved stoically or over-emotionally, or were neglectful or punitive — may have be come a model for in addressing similar situations in the present.

Undue parental attention to childhood illness. If you experienced excessive responses to illness during childhood — toward yourself or others — or if you or others in your family used illness to meet other needs, you may bring these expectations or perceptions into your current pain experience. Doing so can contribute to dysfunctional pain management choices. This is especially true if too much attention and reinforcement was placed on symptoms, suffering, and the role of being sick.

In addition to the above, if you've been diagnosed with one or more of the following mental health issues, either in the past or currently, they will affect your experience of pain and your ability to cope:

- Hypochondria, somatization disorder, or conversion disorder (which all involve either an incorrect or exaggerated sense of injury or disease or misleading, confusing, and sometimes emotionally generated symptoms)
- Hysteria, schizoid personality disorder, dissociative disorder, or emotional repression (all of which involve dysfunctional ways of coping with the anxiety and anger that can result from threats to your needs)

Certain personal orientations can also put you more at risk for dysfunctional approaches to chronic pain:

A sense of being a victim. If you tend to see yourself as a victim whenever you experience physical or emotional pain, this will be disempowering to you and socially off-putting to others.

Trust issues. If, based on childhood experiences, you have difficulty trusting people, this can often be triggered and exacerbated by all the challenges experienced in pain treatment (read more about these challenges in part 4).

Social isolation. If you tend to isolate when you're in distress, this can exacerbate your sense of alienation and loss and reduce the possibility of gaining critically needed support.

Excessive self-reliance. If, based on early experiences, or on too many disappointments in relying on others, you rely excessively on yourself when facing difficulties, you will lose critically needed help and support. Unreasonable and unwarranted rejection of needed help from others is the likely manifestation of this.

Excessive self-sacrifice. If you are in the habit of sacrificing your needs at an extreme level, as a matter of values or habit, you will find it difficult to know what you need or be able to ask for it. Properly managing chronic pain requires that you ask for more — not give more.

And here are a few situational risk factors that can affect pain perception and coping:

Your pain has no obvious relation to injury. This situation can heighten your fear of your pain, activity, rehabilitation, and reinjury.

It's a first-time injury or chronic condition. First-time injuries can reveal your physical vulnerability and mortality, which can heighten your sense of trauma.

You are somatically overfocused. If you're so focused on what's going on physically that you ignore other life impacts and collateral damages, you'll be ignoring the very factors that must be addressed to achieve recovery and thriving.

You've taken on the "sick" role. This situation involves increasing your dependence, passivity, and disempowerment to get the help you need.

You're engaged in disability and/or pain behaviors. In this situation, you display behaviors and communications that exaggerate your pain, either consciously or unconsciously, as a way of seeking help for your pain.

You're homebound. If you allow yourself to become homebound unnecessarily, it will further limit your exposure to positive and empowering activities and encounters that can help in your recovery.

DEPRESSION

The occurrence of some level of depression is not unusual with chronic pain, especially if you don't yet have any sense of power to manage your pain. Feeling helpless and hopeless are part of this experience. Pain and depression can create a vicious cycle in which pain worsens the symptoms of depression, and then the resulting depression worsens the pain.

> "The central component of depression is a defensive reaction to extreme stress — the exact kind of extreme stress that chronic pain can create."

Pain and its impacts can wear you down over time. The loss of physical comfort and functioning caused by pain threatens your needs and stirs up massive amounts of anxiety and anger in reaction. When you recognize that you carry unresolving pain each moment of the day, it's easy to understand how you might lose joy, satisfaction, and contentment. This emotional struggle can — but does not have to — lead to depression. Most people are unaware that depression is not just a medical issue. The central component of depression is a defensive reaction to extreme stress — the exact kind of extreme stress that chronic pain can create. (This will be discussed more in this chapter's Recovery section.)

Depression can include any or all of the following symptoms:

- Feeling very unhappy and sad
- Irritability
- Guilt
- Loss of interest in activities
- Social withdrawal
- Suicidal thoughts
- Poor concentration
- Poor memory
- Indecision
- Slow thinking
- Loss of motivation
- Sleep disturbance, insomnia, hypersomnia
- Appetite disturbance, weight loss or gain
- Fatigue
- Headaches
- Constipation

It's not hard to see how these symptoms can compound a pain problem, both physically and emotionally. Depression can also have negative impacts on the immune system, which undermines healing, and on all aspects of functioning. The more severe the depression, the more significant the impact.

POST-TRAUMATIC STRESS DISORDER (PTSD)

Once called shell shock or battle fatigue syndrome, PTSD is a serious condition that can develop after a person has experienced or witnessed a traumatic event. It is best treated with a combination of both medication and therapy.

Personal vulnerabilities — including prior exposure to traumatic events, one's age at the time of exposure, family instability, lack of social support, major life stressors, ineffective coping mechanisms, poor self-image, and negative values such as cynicism, alienation, and self-doubt — can contribute to the development of PTSD. Any psychosocial factor or personal characteristic can significantly influence the impact that a traumatic event has on your life.

Pain and PTSD are often related. Reexperiencing pain symptoms and dysfunction over and over, and believing you are helpless, can increase the likelihood that, at some point, your pain will become traumatic. Many people with chronic pain meet the criteria for PTSD. And people with PTSD symptoms report higher levels of pain, life interference, emotional distress, and anxiety and anger. Here are some specific factors that contribute to the mutual maintenance of chronic pain and PTSD:

- People with chronic pain and people with PTSD may attend to threatening or painful stimuli with the same level of exaggerated alarm (also called attentional bias).
- People with chronic pain and people with PTSD both catastrophize — or focus on all the worst possible outcomes — when thinking about events.
- Repetitive pain and PTSD may trigger each other, causing avoidance behaviors regarding the cause of pain and any memories of the trauma.
- Fatigue and lethargy may contribute to both pain and PTSD.
- General anxiety may contribute to both pain and PTSD.
- Both pain and PTSD contribute to cognitive impairments that can limit the use of adaptive coping strategies.

Unrelenting, incurable pain creates increasing emotional impact, especially if you don't process your feelings about it. If you suppress the anxiety and anger that arise in response to the impacts of your pain, you'll likely become more afraid of pain and other physical sensations. Habits of avoiding anxiety and anger, as in depression, may also contribute to the development of PTSD.

Unresolved stress and pain that you don't understand will also cause a high degree of alarm and dysfunction and can contribute to PTSD. In turn, PTSD that arose from events prior to one's chronic pain can contribute to habits of avoidance. Avoiding your emotions makes it harder for you to challenge false pain-related beliefs and expectations. Avoidance also keeps you from engaging in activities and social situations that are positive and helpful.

This combination of PTSD and learned avoidance exacerbates the experience of pain. It can lead to heightened arousal, where adrenaline is coursing through your physical system and activating your muscles, causing increased blood flow, rising heart rate, and greater muscle tension. These in turn directly increase sensations of pain and reinforce fears and negative beliefs — it becomes a negative feedback loop. Meanwhile, all these sensations of arousal can be misinterpreted as being related to your pain and add to the creation of PTSD.

PTSD and chronic pain are both likely to exaggerate your sense of being vulnerable — physically, psychologically, and emotionally. People with both PTSD and chronic pain often believe that pain and their emotional reaction to it are both unpredictable and uncontrollable. This perceived lack of control over your pain will add to feelings of helplessness and more trauma.

A belief that you are constantly vulnerable to unpredictable pain and suffering often precedes the development of both chronic pain and PTSD.

PANIC ATTACKS

Panic attacks are not uncommon with chronic pain. A panic attack is an episode of sudden intense fear or anxiety, with physical symptoms, that is based on a perceived threat rather than on an actual imminent danger. Many factors can contribute to panic attacks, including genetics, neurochemical dysfunction, chronic hyperventilation, a respiratory condition called carbon dioxide receptor hypersensitivity, seizure disorders, heightened sensitivity to internal autonomic cues, emotional repression or suppression, and/or faulty patterns of thinking. If you're not aware of how much your chronic pain affects you, or if you suppress your feelings, it's more likely you'll have a panic attack. No matter the cause, panic attacks are disabling and make the management of chronic pain more difficult.

Catastrophizing is a common form of thought distortion that exaggerates the threats of chronic pain and leads you into worst-case-scenario thinking. Because catastrophizing increases your fear of pain, it leads to a variety of reactions: avoidance of activities that may elicit pain, guarding behaviors, and hypervigilance to bodily sensations. Catastrophizing is a significant predictor of negative outcomes for patients with pain and may move you toward panic attacks. Panic attacks contribute to a loss of function and a greater sense of helplessness that fuels your sense of threat even further. The symbiotic relationship between catastrophizing and panic attacks can drive you toward a level of alarm too intense for coherent functioning, and thus another panic attack.

ANXIETY DISORDERS

Anxiety is a normal human emotion with a physical reaction that can help us take action to protect ourselves. When needs arise that can't be addressed or met, the nervous system can be triggered into a heightened state of alarm, part of the fight-or-flight response. This biological response, helpful in the face of actual threat, prepares you for action. It's a powerful response that alters your emotional, mental, and physical state to increase your capacity for action so you can meet the challenge and put the threats to rest. But when a threat to needs is unmet and action cannot immediately be taken, an anxiety disorder may arise. Here's how the cycle often works:

Emotions are activated. These are a few of the emotional states commonly associated with anxiety:

- Apprehension
- Alarm
- Tension/uptightness
- Unease
- Uncertainty or doubt
- Helplessness

Negative mental states are triggered, such as these thought patterns likely to emerge in anxiety:

- Worry (perseveration, obsessing)
- Hypervigilance (increased focus on possible dangers/consequences)
- Catastrophizing (thinking about worst-case scenarios)

These emotional and mental states can then lead to these physical changes:

- Muscle tension
- Increased perspiration
- Increased heart rate and blood pressure
- Gastrointestinal urgency, followed by an upset stomach
- Increased energy and even shakiness
- Cold hands and feet

When experiencing these physical changes, people tend to engage in a set of specific behaviors:

- Restlessness
- Avoidance — particularly of the activities related to the potential danger
- Restricting or avoiding all activities outside of one's home
- Lack of motivation and resistance to completing activities or projects

When anxiety becomes persistent and impairing, it's considered no longer functional but rather improperly used. The nervous system becomes stuck in a persistent state of reactivity, and one's emotional and physical states begin to reshape the nervous system. This is called central sensitization.

Anxiety disorders often accompany chronic pain. There are at least five common types. We have already discussed panic attacks and PTSD. The other three types are generalized anxiety (persistent worry), social anxiety (overwhelming anxiety in everyday social interactions), and obsessive-compulsive disorder (repeated thoughts or rituals that interfere with daily life).

It is common for these five different types of anxiety disorders to occur in combination with each other and with depression. These disorders are correlated with significantly worse pain experiences and diminished health-related quality of life compared with people who have chronic pain but do not have anxiety disorders.

In the presence of chronic pain and its negative impacts, anxiety might very well be expected. It becomes a disorder when it perpetuates a chronic sense of alarm or distress and a constant focus on pain. This leads to chronic muscle tension, which leads to more pain. If, as a person in pain, you try to avoid your chronic anxiety — rather than address it directly — you will add to your sense of social isolation, inactivity, and powerlessness. Ultimately, you will feel more disabled.

ANGER

Anger is an emotion, a form of energy that involves heightened focus and power, and a tool to help you cope. Anger is evoked when anxiety alerts you to threats to your needs. We often think of yelling, screaming, and hitting as anger itself. But these behaviors are not anger; they are a misuse of the energy behind anger. When properly channeled and directed, anger can help you reduce or eliminate the threats to your needs.

Anger is a common emotion experienced in chronic pain — and given all the threats to your needs, how could it not be? However, when anger is mismanaged, you lose your own power to address your needs and manage your pain. Then you may become angry at your pain, your life, your own body, your limitations, and others' actions and attitudes. Anger is not a thing, a place, or a state that you want to reside in. It is something to use — appropriately and effectively. Anger used improperly can and will undermine constructive thinking, creativity, and a focus on solutions. It will negatively affect your physical health, your self-esteem, and your relationships with others. Most important, it will hinder the possibility of recovery.

CHRONIC UNHEALTHY STRESS

Stress is not an emotion. It is not something to get rid of. Healthy stress is the type of stress when you feel excited. In this event, your pulse quickens, your hormones surge, but there is no threat or fear. In its unhealthy manifestation, it is a state of psychological, emotional, and physical imbalance. What triggers this state is the emergence of significant and/or numerous threats to your needs. Given chronic pain's negative impact on multiple human needs, it's not surprising that people with chronic pain experience stress on a chronic basis as well.

The experience of stress is often described as feeling overwhelmed and flooded by worry, anxiety, frustration, and anger. This experience is accompanied by predictable negative changes on your biochemistry, physiology, emotions, psychology, and behavior. Extreme stress will adversely affect many systems of the body, including the immune system, cardiovascular system, neuroendocrine system, and central nervous system. It keeps your fight-or-flight response turned on and in hyperdrive.

Stress takes a great toll on your physical and emotional energy. It also takes a severe toll on your personal psychological power, making you more inclined to feel helpless and hopeless. This is especially true when stress is constant and persists over an extended period. These impacts, in turn, undermine your ability to heal as well as to cope. Simply put, chronic stress, inadequately managed, increases pain and undermines recovery. Resolving stress is central to the work I do with all my patients.

How do you know if you are experiencing chronic stress? There are many potential signs and symptoms, from psychobiological symptoms (such as muscle tension or digestive upset) to cognitive, emotional, and behavioral reactions. Read through the signs and symptoms in table 1 below, and consider how many fit your experience, and how best to address them.

Table 1. Signs of Stress

Psychobiological	Behavioral
Sleep disturbance (insomnia, sleeping fitfully) Clenched jaw, grinding teeth Digestive upsets Lump in your throat Difficulty swallowing Increased heart rate General restlessness Sense of muscle tension body, or actual muscle twitching Noncardiac chest pains Dizziness, lightheadedness Hyperventilation Sweaty palms Nervousness Stumbling over words High blood pressure Lack of energy Fatigue	Decreased contact with family and friends Poor relationships at work Sense of loneliness Decreased sex drive Avoiding others (and being avoided) because you're cranky Failing to set aside time for relaxation through activities such as hobbies, music, art, or reading Substance abuse Agitated behavior, such as twiddling your fingers Playing with your hair
Emotional	Cognitive
Irritation Loss of your sense of humor Frustration Jumpiness, overexcitability Feeling overworked Feeling overwhelmed Sense of helplessness or apathy Sense that life is overwhelming	Mental slowness Confusion General negative attitudes or thinking Constant worry Racing mind Difficulty concentrating Forgetfulness Difficulty thinking in a logical sequence Difficulties with problem-solving

RECOVERY: MENTAL HEALTH AWARENESS

Much can be done to avoid new mental health difficulties being brought on by your chronic pain, to work safely with existing mental health challenges, and to support your recovery from chronic pain. Key to this process are self-knowledge and appropriate support. Even more important is viewing emerging mental health symptoms not as problems but as pointers toward what you need and what solutions to look for. Here are some useful strategies.

Know Your Risk Factors

I can't emphasize enough how important it is that you, your providers, and your supportive others all become aware of the risk factors and historical influences in your life. Your history affects how you experience pain, as well as how you understand it, communicate about it, and cope with it. The childhood risk factors discussed at the beginning of this chapter (loss, abuse, trauma, etc.) have all been shown to influence a person's experience of pain and response to treatment.

So, just like with other impacts, these influences need to be factored in to your awareness and your treatment plan. Each must be explored, processed, and treated as part of your overall recovery. In this regard, chronic pain can be a clearinghouse for the various habits, attitudes, and beliefs that undermine your ability to obtain optimal self-care and support. These influences underscore important aspects of your individual uniqueness that will affect your recovery one way or the other. Typically, mental health history and risk factors are addressed in counseling, but all of your providers need to be aware of and attentive to them. The medical system changes slowly, but patient awareness and demand gradually help to change policy. See part 4 for more specifics on how to engage in this.

Find and Work with the Purpose in Your Depression

Most people treat depression as just another illness, with no meaning other than the suffering it produces. However, from an existential point of view, depression can be understood as an attempt to cope with pain's collateral damages, including the resulting anxiety and anger. From this point of view, depression has a functional purpose. It is a coping mechanism. Chronic pain can cause a tsunami's worth of negative emotions, often way too much to cope with by ordinary means. So, depression — by cutting you off from your feelings — can effectively help you cope in the short term. The moment this happens, of course, is usually not something you'd be consciously aware of.

Unfortunately, the side effects (symptoms) of depression far outweigh any benefit it might offer. You need your feelings. The more accessible they are, and the more you learn to manage and use them effectively and constructively, the more likely it is that you'll be able to prevent or improve your depression *and* your pain.

In addition to working with feelings, there are several traditional approaches to treating depression. Antidepressant medications can help relieve pain by addressing the balance of chemicals in the brain, in partic-ular the levels of serotonin and norepineph-rine. Medication combined with various forms of counseling can be very effective. One form of individual therapy for depression that is very effective on its own is cognitive-behav-ioral therapy. The goal of cognitive-behavioral therapy is to change your mood and experi-ence of life by identifying negative and distorted thinking patterns. This form of therapy emphasizes the link between thoughts, feelings, and behavior. It helps identify the way that certain thoughts contribute to the unique problems of your life. By chang-ing the thought pattern, both feelings and behavior will change, which in turn can reduce depression.

> "The solution will be in your willingness to acknowledge and embrace the anxiety and anger, using them to teach you about your losses and needs."

If you are not drawn to individual therapy, you might consider partic-ipating in group therapy. There are many pain rehabilitation programs, such as the comprehensive Pain Rehabilitation Center at the University of Washington and one at the Mayo Clinic, which typically provide a team approach to treatment, including both medical and psychiatric approaches.

Treatment for co-occurring pain and depression may be most effective when it involves a combination of treatments. Stress-reduction techniques, physical activity, exercise, meditation, journaling, learning coping skills, and other strategies may all help. Ultimately, the solution will be in your willingness to acknowledge and embrace the anxiety and anger that chronic pain creates — not shutting them down but using them to teach you about your losses and needs. In this way, you can eliminate dysfunc-tional coping mechanisms and instead use the positive abilities you were endowed with as a human being.

Address PTSD with Self-Knowledge

The most important factor in preventing or recovering from PTSD is to appreciate that PTSD, like depression, is your psyche's way of coping with overwhelming anxiety caused by a perceived major threat to your needs. PTSD acts to block and contain the threat. PTSD is very difficult to manage or recover from.

There are things you can do that can reduce your likelihood of developing PTSD, reduce the intensity of your PTSD, or resolve PTSD if you have already experienced it. The essential tools are ones we have discussed many times already:

- Become more aware that we, as humans, are all vulnerable. There are many events and experience in life that can harm us emotionally, physically, and psychologically. If you are aware of this, you can do many things to prevent, prepare, and cope with them successfully.
- Get to know yourself in detail, with patience, self-compassion, and support. Self-transformation can take you from surviving to thriving, and it starts right here.
- Learn more constructive ways to process your anxiety and anger.
- Explore a wide range of coping styles, beliefs, expectations, patterns of emotional regulation, and self-awareness.

If you have PTSD already, your treatment needs to help you feel safe enough to acknowledge and process the feelings that are locked down. You can support this path by developing your ability to experience and process anxiety constructively, as described in various sections in this book.

Some drugs used to alleviate pain may have a secondary benefit of preventing or treating PTSD.

PTSD also responds well to different forms of cognitive-behavioral therapy. In this work, you can experience both *situational exposure* exercises (such as doing activities that you previously avoided) as well as *interoceptive exposure* exercises (such as spinning in a chair or running in place), which are designed to help you identify, face, and cope with uncomfortable inner bodily sensations.

More than anything, you need to understand that you can act now to prevent additional trauma from your chronic pain. The more effectively you understand your needs and act to meet or restore satisfaction of your needs, the less likely your pain will evolve into PTSD.

Reduce Panic by Increasing Awareness

Panic attacks are an expression of suppressed feelings. As with other mental health disturbances, panic attacks are a form of coping that have side effects that are worse than the benefit. They cause an increased sense of vulnerability and helplessness.

> "You can avoid panic attacks by addressing the threats to your needs."

Counseling and medication are the typical approaches to dealing with panic attacks and catastrophic thinking. Both can be helpful. In the approach I advocate in this book, you can avoid panic attacks by addressing the threats to your needs caused by pain and learning various cognitive coping strategies to manage them successfully. When you learn to express the negative emotions you feel in reaction to those threats, and to process them, you will be generally less anxious, and less likely to have a panic attack. These approaches can be learned in counseling and then self-maintained.

You can also learn to confront catastrophic thinking, or exaggeration of the danger in your pain. Your commitment to learning to be more comfortable with being vulnerable, strengthened through therapy, will empower you to better address your challenges. Eventually, it will become habit for you to examine the truth of your condition, and then consider all the means and ways you might reduce the extent of pain's impact on you and increase your functioning. As you develop these capabilities, you'll be less likely to experience panic attacks or catastrophic thinking. Understand that your negative emotions exist to serve your needs by guiding your choices. Once you know this, negative emotions are less likely to overwhelm you.

Reduce Anxiety by Increasing Awareness

Anxiety is a warning system that alerts you to a threat to your needs. It is not something that arises because you are shameful or weak. It's more than a feeling or experience; it can be a tool to help you cope. The more you learn about this emotion and how to manage it, through cognitive-behavioral therapy or other counseling approaches, the better use you will make of it and the less disabling it will be.

Anxiety often demands that you acknowledge painful, negative, and frightening realities, and you will need help in doing this. But if you can accomplish this, you will be able to tap into your internal knowledge and wisdom as well as receive the aid of others who can help you minimize the threats in your life. You may also benefit from participating in a pain management program, especially one with a rehabilitation and recovery orientation. Such programs help to reduce any sense of threat from pain.

Learn How Anger Can Serve You

There really are no anger management issues, only anger *mis*management issues. As you become more aware of the consequences of your choices, you will want to learn the skills to use anger constructively. Anger can and should be used to find ways to reduce the threats to your needs and to help motivate positive and constructive changes in your condition and your ability to function. Used properly, anger will fuel your empowerment. It will help offset the damage to your life that chronic pain creates. Counseling is the appropriate venue in which to address this.

Prevent Chronic Stress

Everyday stressors can be managed with healthy stress management behaviors, which are outlined in detail in chapter 9. But chronic stress requires a unique set of coping and management skills, which begin with understanding what stress is. Stress is a psychobiological state created by a threat or threats to fundamental human needs, such as a job, a home, relationships, life. When we are flooded by anxiety and anger in response to these threats, a psychobiological imbalance occurs. Managing these naturally occurring emotions, as described in all the previous Recovery sections in this chapter, will restore that balance and prevent stress from becoming chronic. You can also break the pattern of chronic stress by utilizing the principles and practices in this book.

This chapter brings to a close our examination of most of the experiences and impacts that chronic pain can bring on both the physical and personal levels, and the various recovery techniques that are available. In the two chapters in part 4, we turn our focus to the treatment environment and the obstacles — both external and internal — it poses to people living with chronic pain.

Tools and Takeaways for Part 4

The two chapters in part 4 outline the challenges (chapter 17) and recovery strategies (chapter 18) pertinent to the treatment environment for people seeking relief and healing from chronic pain. The self-assessment inventories in appendix C can help you identify which treatment-related impacts are most relevant to you:

- Treatment Confusion Inventory
- Treatment Experience Inventory
- Treatment Visit Evaluation Inventory

Bottom Line

Information and communication are at the heart of a successful treatment experience. Your providers and consultants work for you and are the experts in their fields. But you are the expert on your needs and experience, and you can use your holistic knowledge , tools, attitudes, and strategies to develop deeper and more productive partnerships with your providers.

PART 4

The Treatment
Experience

Chapter 17

Challenges in the Treatment Environment

The existential model that informs this book recognizes *all* the collateral damages from chronic pain. Perhaps surprisingly, these damages include those that arise from pain treatment and treatment plans. The goal of this chapter is to help you understand the potential obstacles that are inherent in the treatment environment, including the limitations in treatment models that have, unfortunately, shaped so many treatment protocols throughout the medical and insurance industries.

With this chapter's focus on the treatment environment, you'll begin to see what might be achieved with a deeper understanding of what you need from your plan and your providers. It will begin to highlight some of the ways you (and your providers) can use the existential, holistic approach laid out in this book to add great value and success to your treatment experience.

Though this whole chapter focuses on obstacles, don't lose heart! It gives you foundational information for chapter 18, which will provide immense practical help in how to successfully navigate the treatment environment. You will emerge from part 4 with a wealth of tools, attitudes, and strategies to guide you in becoming an empowered, proactive patient. Most importantly, the goal of these two chapters together is to help you develop deeper and more productive partnerships with your providers.

OBSTACLES IN THE TREATMENT ENVIRONMENT

The traditional pain treatment model limits its scope to alleviation of symptoms and curing the initial injury or disease that gave rise to your chronic pain. It presupposes that once your initial injury or disease has been dealt with, you should be fine; in this model, collateral damages are not well assessed or considered.

Not surprisingly, then, most obstacles in chronic pain treatment fall broadly under the categories of lack of information, communication problems, and mistaken expectations. These themselves are related to limited time and access to providers in the traditional model. Incomplete, inadequate, ambiguous, or confusing information is at the heart of unsuccessful treatment. You may also bring your own obstacles to treatment success into the treatment environment — such as guardedness, shyness, aversion to conflict, or disorganization. Habits and behaviors like these make it difficult to forge a fruitful collaboration with your provider.

> "Remember, you are the expert on your pain experience."

Whatever your experiences in treatment have been, remember that any problems you may have encountered point to the importance of the quality of your interactions with your providers. Reflecting on these interactions will help underscore the importance of having and providing *complete* information. As you read through this chapter, consider how such information could empower you and your providers. Remember, *you* are the expert on your pain experience.

What is considered complete, clear, and relevant information to be exchanged in medical treatment? The answer is in the holistic, multi-dimensional model for understanding chronic pain that this book has outlined so far. The first part of a successful communication process originates with you — with your thorough explanation of your situation, including your physical pain, injury, and questions concerning what exactly is causing you chronic pain. The second part involves the provider explaining to you how their recommended treatment interventions will help to reduce or eliminate your pain. Two halves of a full understanding.

Adequate information leads to more accurate expectations. You and your providers both need to receive information that is thorough and accurate so you both have reasonable expectations for how much your pain can be reduced, what level of functioning can be recovered, and how long it is likely to take.

I introduced you to Michelle in chapter 1. Michelle was suffering from an increasingly disabling shoulder injury. From her first doctor's visit through appointments with the specialists that followed, she craved information. More than anything, she just wanted to understand the basics:

- What is the structural nature of my injury?
- Why is it continuing to cause pain?
- What can be done to treat it?

She wanted specific information, that she could understand, about how much treatment was recommended, for how long, and what she could expect from it. She was operating from a simple premise: "It hurts, I'm broken, fix me." She thought the advice her providers would give her would be similarly simple, direct, and straightforward.

> "Adequate information leads to more accurate expectations."

Indeed, Michelle's providers also started from a simple premise: Working from the (extremely limited) traditional model of chronic pain, they expected to fix the original problem; job done. But the impact of pain on Michelle's overall functioning was at odds with everyone's expectations.

Michelle's expectation of a simple explanation and cure were not met. Her pain was not significantly relieved, and her normal functioning was not restored. Not only that, but Michelle did not gain from her providers any clear explanation of why her treatment had failed.

This is a good example of how a lack of understanding and information can deepen the negative impact on someone's recovery. Had Michelle's providers started with full information from an existential, holistic approach like the one discussed in this book, her treatment plan and its outcomes could have been much more positive. Unfortunately, that did not happen.

For Michelle and her providers, it was like reading a story that starts in chapter three, with half the characters and plot for the book missing! Because her providers failed to understand the totality of what contributed to Michelle's pain, they came to incorrect conclusions, and Michelle experienced increased anxiety and anger. By the time I met her, she was depressed and feeling helpless and hopeless. She believed she was disabled. Her providers weren't sure they could help her. Michelle and her medical providers had experienced a shared journey — from an acute condition to one of ongoing suffering — utterly without understanding what had happened.

This not only resulted in an extremely limited treatment response, it created a worse prognosis. Michelle had inadvertently become one of the vagabonds of medical care, wandering without clear purpose through the system, beleaguered, stereotyped, her fate seemingly predicted and sealed.

THE STRUCTURE OF TREATMENT

When I met Michelle, we fully analyzed the *total experience* of her pain and how it had impacted her life. This analysis revealed important information that clarified — for Michelle and her providers — all the impacts that affected her injury and treatments, and this information eventually led to a more successful recovery.

Let's look at the elements of communication involved in treatment and the failures that often lie within. The eight sections that follow show how treatment errors commonly begin: with delayed or time-limited access to providers, medical specialization, lack of coordination and integration, communication problems, incorrect beliefs and expectations, burdensome documentation requirements, insurance complications, and treatment errors (see figure 1). Becoming mindful of the potential problems in these areas is important — it allows for the possibility of preventing them, neutralizing them, or minimizing their impact. The skills and methods to do so are explored in detail in the next chapter.

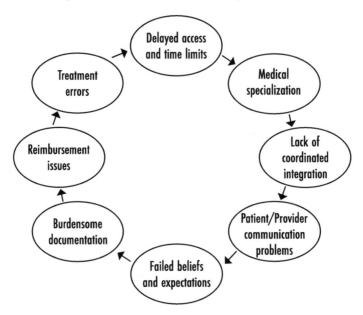

Figure 1. Cycle of Treatment Failures

Delayed Access and Time Limits

Time is of the essence in chronic pain. If it's difficult to get an appointment with your providers, you may not get treatment when you need it. If appointments don't allow enough time for discussion, you may not be able to ask all your questions or get the answers you need.

The amount of time providers dedicate to an appointment is determined by their understanding of your condition, good medical practice, and what they presume you need and want to know. In current practice, it is not unusual for this to average fifteen to twenty minutes of full attention from your provider. In addition, a portion of your appointment time is often handled by a nurse or other assistant whose initial assessment affects the two-way interaction between you and your provider. This brief screening assessment determines what the provider will ask and what information they will give you. In other words, by the time the provider steps into the exam room, they may believe they already have *all* the information they need about your condition!

However, the amount of time spent should be based on actual needs, not presumptions. Without a holistic, existential approach such as that described in this book, it's quite likely that your provider won't be aware of the extent of the impacts from your pain, your feelings about your condition in terms of what it means in your life, or how you feel about treatment. And they may not have scheduled enough time to obtain such an existential, holistic understanding of your chronic pain. You may never get to know your doctors and they may never get to know you.

These time-related limitations in the medical environment are problematic for anyone, but for those who suffer from chronic pain, they can add significantly to the cumulative, unrelenting, and anxiety producing aspects of your pain. Waiting for relief or reassurance can wear you down in a much different way than it would for someone with an acute complaint. And any increase in your anxiety, anger, and distress can amplify your pain. This situation may leave you feeling neglected and uncared for or damage your self-esteem. In between visits, as you wait for your providers to "fix you," you may feel powerless to help yourself or manage your pain.

Another reason that short and infrequent visits are problematic is that it becomes more likely that you won't have a chance to give your providers sufficient information about your situation, including what has happened or is happening to you physically, emotionally, and psychologically. *This situation* limits the opportunity for providers to get to know you as an individual. Your providers may end up with a major lack of information about your identity, values, needs, and personal history, as well as about the long list of emotional, psychological, and life impacts your pain may have caused. All of this is relevant to your condition and treatment.

Omission of this information can, in turn, produce medical documentation that is inadequate, incomplete, or inaccurate. Since each new provider counts on past documentation to familiarize themselves with your case, prior lack of information and documentation compounds future providers' lack of understanding and appreciation of the factors that contribute to your pain. Inadequate documentation, then, can undermine the exploration of possible preventative measures and self-care options that could empower you in your recovery.

Ideally, you would be able to see your providers as frequently as your condition dictated — with adequate time at each visit for them to get to know you and the unique experiences and individual differences that make you who you are, and to think critically about or research the reasons your condition presents as it does.

Here are just a few examples of how important some types of information are for a full understanding of your situation:

Loss. Your pain may have cost you your job, damaged your relationships, or undermined your sense of identity. These experiences are likely quite stressful, and this stress can exacerbate your pain and emotional suffering and undermine your commitment to treatment.

Stoicism. If you're a stoic person who identifies with being tough or is uncomfortable with emotional vulnerability, your past reports may have underrepresented your pain and your functional or emotional impacts.

Past trauma. Some treatments — injections, physical therapy, palpation — come with a bit of pain. If you have suffered prior physical or sexual abuse or other trauma, you may interpret pain, even from beneficial treatment, as abusive or deeply disturbing — without even knowing why. A trauma history can cause strong, hard-to-understand emotional reactions and treatment resistance.

In short, your personal history about pain and suffering is quite important. If you and your providers both know as much relevant history as possible, it can be factored into your treatment and eliminated as a potential contributor to negative impacts.

On the other hand, when a provider lacks knowledge of you as an individual, they may misunderstand even basic information. Take, for example, the standard 0 to 10 pain rating scale. This system rates pain in a global sense, with no objective standard except for past reports, which of course are based on wholly subjective experiences. If providers could focus on pain as it relates to your personal history and functioning, the scale might become more mean-

> "A provider who lacks knowledge of you as an individual may misunderstand even basic information."

ingful. For example, do your providers know or consider if you are, on the one hand, a former athlete, police officer, or Zen master, or, on the other hand, highly sensitive or unaccustomed to strain or injury? A person mentally trained to handle pain will use the scale differently than someone who has never had to deal with pain before, or who is afraid of it. One person's 9 may be another person's 6, or 12!

Does your provider know if you are someone who, even though you have pain, can mostly still function? Or if you can hardly function at all at times? Do they know that with some types of pain histories, physical therapy treatment is more likely to fail if such details are not taken into account?

It's also important for you to obtain relevant information *from* your provider. The absence of sufficient information can cause people not to follow treatment recommendations — a significant safety issue. Here's a personal story I use as an example of the mutual benefits of having more information: I once suffered a herniated disc and had to go through physical therapy. Because of my background in martial arts, I was used to intense training, and I thought the treatment I was being given was not nearly intense enough to help. If I had not asked a lot of questions about the physical therapist's approach, I might have dropped out of treatment and gone my own way. On the other hand, once the therapist knew about my martial arts training, they could use that knowledge to the treatment's advantage.

When your own history and any past discipline and training is understood and respected by a provider, you can use it to enhance your treatment. If, because of confusion or lack of trust, you decide (consciously or otherwise) not to follow the steps of your treatment plan, the result can be more damage and unnecessary disability rather than alleviation of suffering and pain.

Lack of adequate time for information-taking can also generate premature, incorrect, or unnecessary tests and referrals. A limited assessment of your needs can lead providers in early stages of treatment to depend more on outside tests and studies such as X-rays and MRIs. Compared to direct provider examination, many of these tests are more subject to false positives in diagnosis. Relying too heavily on tests may lead to either over-investigation or under-investigation. Further, such an approach is more likely to lead to unnecessary, potentially harmful, and expensive procedures than a recovery-oriented approach would.

As you move from primary care providers to specialists, you begin working with providers who rely even more on the medical reports, test results, and exams provided to them. The test-oriented approach fosters the false notion that people with chronic pain can be "fixed" and over-simplifies the true nature of what is generating the pain. These limits can bias providers as they develop theories about your condition and can lead to incorrect treatment recommendations.

Suppose missed critical information results in inaccurate or limited assessments, mistaken analysis, misdiagnoses or missed diagnoses, or prescription errors. Now you're facing treatment that will cause more harm than help. These situations are potentially devastating to both you and your providers. If your visits had started with complete information on collateral damages and a running commentary from you about additional impacts occurring across time, all these pitfalls could be avoided. This information exchange could be accomplished even within limited treatment time by completing comprehensive pre-submitted assessment forms.

Altogether, the conclusions you and your provider draw in the context of too little information about your collateral damages may lead to underdiagnosis or misdiagnosis and affect access to care. I've seen many cases where the initial diagnosis was mistaken and did not allow for more comprehensive tests such as an MRI or referral to appropriate specialists.

For example, Marie was, at thirty-five years of age, the victim of a slip-and-fall accident that led to severe chronic back pain. Her primary care physician did a traditional examination, with an emphasis on the purely physical aspects of her case. Marie claimed that her pain was increasing and continuing to undermine her functioning. But since her doctor hadn't seen anything significant in her X-rays, he thought she was exaggerating and catastrophizing. He didn't see the need for further studies and instead told her to "take it easy" for a while and take ibuprofen as needed. He scheduled her future appointments across several months.

Eventually, eight months after the original injury, and acknowledging that he was at a loss to explain Marie's continuing complaints of increased pain and dysfunction, her doctor sent her to an acute care sports medicine doctor. That doctor relied on her primary care provider's assessment of "lumbar strain and sprain with patient exaggeration of symptoms" and ordered an intensive course of physical therapy. The physical therapist relied on the two prior physicians' assessments. Unfortunately, as it later turned out, Marie had several herniated discs and radiculopathy, and so was further injured by the physical therapy.

After she came to me, we were able, through our thorough, holistic assessment, to discover and supply the necessary information to Marie's providers. A reactivation plan was developed, and eventually she was successful in her rehabilitation.

Communication breakdowns and unmet expectations can also inhibit recovery. Take the case of Clyde, thirty-four years old and suffering from thoracic outlet syndrome, a nerve-related condition that causes significant chronic pain in the shoulder and neck. This condition is hard to diagnose and hard to treat successfully. Clyde's doctor focused on the medical treatment options, which are few, and believed there was nothing more he could do to help Clyde. Because of this, in the doctor's busy practice, he didn't consider seeing Clyde to be a priority, and so he set Clyde's medical appointments to be six weeks to three months apart. Meanwhile, Clyde was experienced collateral damages, including mounting frustration and anxiety between appointments, due to his limited understanding of his condition. He had lost his job and many of his friends, his marriage was disintegrating, and his coping skills were inadequate to manage the stress. These life impacts could have been addressed had his doctor engaged in a more holistic understanding of Clyde's condition. At the very least, the doctor could have changed Clyde's treatment schedule, which could possibly have prevented or at least minimized these impacts. However, increasing the frequency of Clyde's visits was only accomplished after I assessed his condition, advised his providers, and provided the missing treatment to address Clyde's collateral damages.

As you can see, delayed or limited access to your providers can have major negative consequences for your potential to recover. When the frequency of visits and the time allotted for your care are instead based on an existential and holistic model, it can make each encounter more meaningful and in turn empower you to positively transform your treatment outcomes. This remains true throughout treatment.

Excessive time between visits or inadequate time during visits, on the other hand, can be damaging to your recovery. This becomes apparent once you understand the depth and complexity of the negative impacts your pain has caused. You need for time to *aid* you in recovery, not become part of the problem. Six weeks to several months between provider appointments is often too long: Accumulative damage from chronic pain can occur daily in pain flare-ups and other pain-related crises. You need easy access to providers, not emergency rooms.

> "You need easy access to providers, not emergency rooms."

Waiting sets the stage for all kinds of possible complications. Just as delays in restoring power and safe drinking water after an earthquake can create serious health problems for disaster victims, delaying care for chronic conditions can create additional damage. Delays in care likely mean that treatment encounters will be less productive, less positive, and less motivating. Delays can undermine your trust in your providers, weaken your commitment to treatment, and, worst of all, kill your belief in recovery.

All the problems described in this section revolve around the inadequate traditional assessment model providers work from — as well as constraints in the treatment environment itself. Information and preparation on your part are critical to overcoming potential problems. While your providers may be constrained by the traditional approach in their questions and information-giving, you do not have to be. You can plan for good communication — for example, by preparing a report on your condition, a list of questions, and an agenda for each encounter with your providers. You can research your condition and your treatments to orient yourself and become focused for your meetings and, in doing so, be able to ask good, relevant questions. (We'll discuss these strategies in more detail in chapter 18, "Mastering the Treatment Experience.")

Specialization and Its Limitations

Medical specialists spend most of their schooling focusing on their own areas of specialty. They learn the intricacies of their chosen body system, the diseases and conditions that affect their chosen body system, and the ways to heal their chosen body system — they spend years concentrating on that specialty. After their medical training, they continue learning by reading medical journals that address the same body system, networking with other physicians in their specialty areas, and attending conferences and additional coursework that further their knowledge in their area of specialization.

Though it is likely that your primary care physician (PCP) is your starting point for care when you have an injury or are trying to manage chronic pain, when your pain persists beyond your doctor's expectations, the next step is likely a referral to a specialist. Specialties that are part of chronic pain rehabilitation can include orthopedic interventions, surgeries, physical and occupational therapy, acupuncture, chiropractic, and massage therapy. Other specialties include osteopathy, yoga, tai chi, meditation, naturopathy, and nutrition.

> "Ask your PCP to explain to you, in detail, the logic and potential value in referring you to that specialist."

Which specialists you need to see, in what order (or concurrently), how many visits you need, and how long your treatment will last are questions that will be best addressed if your PCP and specialists are aided by a holistic, existential understanding of pain impacts. This combined approach — a broad and thorough understanding combined with the expertise of one or more specialists — works best when the specialists also can organize and manage chronic pain holistically. For example, orthopedists and surgeons have great value when their services are needed, but their focus is generally limited, and physiatrists (rehabilitation specialists) may be better able to address the bigger picture.

Your PCP, as the medical provider who knows you and your history the best, would be the one expected to quarterback your case. They determine your care plan, which can include tests and referrals — it is reasonable to expect that your PCP knows which specialist or specialists you need.

Ideally, your PCP will be generally knowledgeable about chronic pain management. But they may not be — most PCPs work within a traditional medical approach, which we've repeatedly identified as failing to include important information. Nonetheless, it's important that your PCP stay involved in your case, even if your direct care is taken over by a specialist. Why? Because your PCP's information, even if it is limited, gets passed on to specialists. By definition, specialists will have less general knowledge of you as a person, your pain's impact, and your pain history, medical and otherwise, that can compound problems in diagnosis and treatment.

Before a referral is made, be careful to ask your PCP to explain to you, in detail, the logic and potential value in referring you to that specialist. Consider how the referral aligns with a holistic approach to understanding your problem and successfully treating it. Become informed about the differences in the specialties, in terms of both diagnostic orientation and treatment interventions. Understand that some specialists only specialize in one aspect of the body and don't necessarily learn the intricacies of a body with multiple pain problems — they may not understand chronic pain as a system. This makes error more likely.

Consider the case of Rita, fifty-three years old and experiencing chronic back pain. Rita was injured while working with disabled children. Her PCP diagnosed her with a lumbar sprain, based on X-rays and a cursory examination. Due to his busy practice and office reimbursement issues, his limited knowledge of Rita's life, and his lack of understanding of chronic pain, he failed to assess any other impacts to Rita's life from her pain. He couldn't understand its profound impact on her functioning.

> "Specialists may not understand chronic pain as a system."

Feeling out of his depth, he referred Rita to an orthopedist, a specialist who mostly focused on the mechanical aspects of her pain. Assuming that Rita's PCP had assessed all the relevant data, the orthopedist based his understanding on the PCP's report. He based *his* findings purely on a structural analysis, and so was at odds to explain her condition. He referred her to another specialist, who was equally mystified.

Rita came to me a year and a half into her problem. Because of her pain and functional limitations, she could not work. She had lost her job. Her home was in foreclosure. Her marriage was on the rocks. Her doctor had her thinking, "I must be crazy; he tells me it's all in my head!"

A thorough impact analysis completely dispelled this notion and indicated that there was likely a much more serious structural problem. Based on this assessment, Rita got an MRI, which revealed serious structural issues, including nerve damage and structural instability. This finally led to appropriate treatment, including physical therapy, acupuncture, massage, and pain management counseling focusing on stress management.

Rita's new treatment plan led to an eventual physical recovery; in time, the damage to her life was also repaired successfully.

Some specialists are better suited than Rita's to understanding and treating their clients' problems, but if their assessment model is limited and does not address collateral damage, they may have trouble understanding the scope and extent of the true damage caused by the pain.

Consider Sally, who I first introduced in chapter 10. She had complained of stomach pains for several weeks. She visited her PCP, who referred her to a gastroenterologist — a specialist who takes care of people's digestive systems — everything from the stomach to the intestines to the colon. The gastroenterologist sent Sally for some tests, and when the results came back, he told Sally he didn't see any problems. He prescribed a drug to help control the nausea, and Sally went home, hoping the nausea would go away.

Weeks went by, and Sally's stomach upset continued to get worse.

She returned to the gastroenterologist, who ran more tests but still was not able to identify her problem. She returned to her PCP, who couldn't find anything either. Neither doctor knew Sally very well, and each assumed the symptoms could be related to stress and anxiety related to her high-responsibility corporate job.

When Sally began to dehydrate from vomiting, her husband took her to the emergency room. A CT scan revealed ovarian cancer. Her PCP had missed it. Her gastroenterologist had missed it. Both were focused on the digestive system and stomach upset, and hadn't considered a problem that might stem from Sally's reproductive system. Fortunately, Sally received the needed treatment and survived.

But how did this happen?

Because they concentrate so completely on their one body system, specialists may not learn the intricacies of how other body systems work or how they interact with one another. If someone presents with familiar-to-their-specialty symptoms but they cannot figure out the problem, they often don't think to send that person to a different specialist.

Most of us assume that our doctors learned all the general information they needed before they specialized. Some do, but not all. Often, it is that lack of general knowledge that stands between a patient and a true diagnosis. In Sally's case, her true medical problem would have been accurately diagnosed by a gynecologist, but neither her PCP nor her gastroenterologist realized they needed to send her to one. The system of assessment they used did not include enough information about Sally or her experience.

Lack of Coordination and Integration

People with chronic pain consistently report that they don't know who's in charge of their treatment or how it all goes together to help them.

The traditional medical system works best with acute or readily identifiable problems such as a broken arm, pneumonia, or gallstones. Many medical providers have limited understanding of what causes and sustains persistent pain. Primary care physicians and specialists alike often lack experience in long-term pain and symptom management, or care and rehabilitation for chronic pain. Furthermore, communication and coordination of care between your primary care provider and specialists may be lacking. They often do not work in the same practice group. They may not share the same model for treatment or share an agreed-upon understanding of what causes chronic pain.

Like other medical conditions, chronic pain is best met with a multi-disciplinary team approach to care, which includes various specialists. It's important to determine which provider is best suited to manage this, because care coordination plays a major role in the quality of your care and positive outcomes.

> "Care coordination plays a major role in the quality of your care and outcomes."

If your doctors can agree on a holistic existential approach to pain management, that common understanding can help them coordinate and integrate your care, making it easier for them to communicate and be on the same page in helping you.

You may expect your primary care doctor or other attending doctor to have reviewed all your previous medical records; consulted with your other providers, past and present; and reviewed all your studies and treatments. For many reasons, however, this may not be the case, and you may be left in search of who is in charge. In your personal crisis, you may not have any appropriately trained medical professional to manage the continuity in your care.

An example of this situation occurred when I was working at the state psychiatric center treating chronic mental illness. When I started, I thought all I needed to know was the proper counseling techniques to help my patients. I soon discovered that this was not enough. Instead, counseling was central to building a working relationship with my patients so we could attain the real goal — of rehabilitating their lives. To do this, I had to learn about social work, case management, psychiatry, medicine, and psychiatric rehabilitation, all organized toward recovery.

General practitioners may not have the time or experience to effectively manage chronic pain; specialists know their specialties best and are not coordinating overall care. But as we've mentioned throughout this book, the real problem lies in the limited conceptual model both are using.

Even current rehabilitation specialists and chronic pain programs, while better grounded conceptually in managing chronic pain, do not have the complete perspective described here. They lack the approach they need to integrate and coordinate the various treatment interventions.

The result is that you may experience treatment as a relay race with no optimal outcomes or good end. As you move through treatment unsuccessfully, you may even find that your care providers seem to be looking to hand off responsibility for your case to the next provider in line. You may keep searching for the "right provider." Ironically, my clients often say that I'm the first provider who they feel "gets" their problem and can make sense of all the other treatments they receive, giving them some hope of a road to recovery.

Communication Failures

Remember, this section — like others in this chapter — is meant to point out what *could* go wrong in treatment. It is not meant to suggest that the problems described here are the typical or likely experience.

All human communication comes with a range of possible outcomes: those that are constructive, connecting, and even enlightening, and those that are non-constructive, disconnected, and confusing. In my practice with chronic pain clients, many say it takes only seconds from the start of a meeting with their doctor before the doctor interrupts, side-tracking them from saying what they need to say and from conveying what the doctor needs to know.

Whether before, during, or after diagnosis or treatment, how often is your doctor clear about what is happening now and what will happen next? How often are your questions answered? Does your doctor help you understand what is going on immediately, and what your outcomes might be? If your doctor is sending you for a medical test, are you told what the expected results or outcomes might be and what they would mean? If not, you'll have less confidence about the process. My experience over the last twenty years has demonstrated that effective doctor-patient communication can make a major difference in all objective measures of recovery.

> "Effective doctor-patient communication can make a major difference in all objective measures of recovery."

Without a holistic existential perspective on your treatment needs, you may not know which questions to ask your doctor, and which to save for others. You may not know how to do it successfully in a limited amount of time. Most of us are not trained or coached in asking questions or in what information is relevant about our conditions that should be shared.

I often suggest that all questions should flow from whatever it is about your condition that makes you anxious. It may be hard for you to know what is appropriate to share with your doctor, other than the usual pain report. For example, how important are your feelings about treatment? How anxious are you about your condition? Should your overall suffering be part of the conversation? And while you might expect communication to be less of an issue for your doctors, as trained professionals, they too have communication limitations.

Here are some of the most common patient-provider communication problems:

Inadequate information gathering. Doctors often pursue a closed, "doctor-centered" approach to information gathering that may unintentionally discourage you from telling the entire story of your chronic pain experience or discussing all of the damage to you and your life. Many providers use closed questions (limited to yes/no answers) as well as lengthy, multiple, and repetitive questions. (Open questions prompt substantially more relevant information.) Doctors learned this style at medical school, but it can produce a premature focus on the purely medical part of your problem. This can limit your ability to communicate your concerns and lead to an overly narrow approach to understanding what is causing your pain. Which in turn will lead to inaccurate consultations, diagnoses, or referrals.

> "Doctors use a communication style taught at medical school, which can produce a premature focus on the purely medical part of your problem."

My experience with clients with chronic pain over the last two decades has also frequently revealed serious limitations in some providers' information-gathering skills. Without good information-gathering skills, these providers are unable to elicit the impact of a patient's pain on daily life, respond to verbal cues, explore ambiguous statements or more personal topics, or use communication to make it easier for their patients to be more forthcoming. This inhibits doctors' abilities to clarify the exact nature of the problem.

For example, providers may not consider racial, gender, cultural, language, or age differences. They may not explicitly ask about your knowledge, beliefs, concerns, and attitudes about your pain. With the best of intensions, they may nonetheless evade discussion of your ideas when you spontaneously bring them up. I would estimate that most providers do not elicit more than 50 percent of the critically important information they need to successfully manage someone's care.

Also, providers may fail to use attentive listening, thus discouraging patients from disclosing significant concerns or psychosocial problems and from expressing their emotions. Providers often don't establish eye contact in a way that's likely to detect emotional distress, nor are they necessarily trained in emotion-handling skills.

In fact, some providers are inclined to remind you that *they're* the doctor and the expert on all aspects of your pain and treatment. They may disagree not just about your pain but about the influence of psychosocial problems on your pain. In several situations, I've known providers to interrupt patients so soon after they begin their opening statement that those patients then fail to share significant concerns and needs. Doctors may also interrupt patients *after* the initial expressed concern, apparently assuming that the first complaint is the chief one. Yet people don't always present their problems in order of importance.

Inadequate understanding of the patient's perspective. You hold valuable and often critical information relevant to helping you recover. Unfortunately, if your providers have limited communication skills or are caught in a narrow focus on your injury, they may not ask you to volunteer all of your experience, even of major life impacts and concerns. Even well-meaning providers may evade statements or questions about these topics or inhibit your expression if you do offer this information. Sometimes there is a discordance between providers' information and your own information and beliefs about your pain. If this gap remains, the end result is likely to be poor understanding, poor adherence to treatment (on your part), and poor outcomes.

Underexplaining or overexplaining. You should be able to expect a full explanation about everything concerning your chronic pain. Unfortunately, providers may underestimate your need and desire for information in many of your encounters. Years of experience have also shown me that most people with chronic pain underestimate their own need for information as well.

Lack of information not only creates problems in recovery, it also causes additional stress. You need optimal and extensive understanding of your pain and treatment experience. There is no doubt that with enough information, your stress will lower significantly, and you will be more likely to recover.

It may be difficult for your providers — and you — to remember that you are treating not just your physical pain but your emotional and psychological pain as well. In a circular fashion, the stress of this then increases the pain. In my experience, controlling stress levels can lead to experiencing a 20 to 30 percent reduction in pain, even when the physical condition has not changed. I often work with clients and providers who are inadequately informed, and it is shocking to me that they don't understand or recognize that information has the power to lead to recovery.

Do you and your providers have a shared way of understanding your pain and treatment needs? How much do interpersonal and situational factors interfere with good communication? There may be vocabulary differences, different educational and social factors, different communication abilities and styles. Doctors may use words and concepts you do not understand. They are trained to use a baffling lexicon of med-speak. Some general medical terms are used by all doctors and many specialties; other words and concepts are specific to body systems, conditions, diseases, or treatments. In many cases, not having learned what you need to know, you may walk away confused and unsatisfied with your visit.

Do you stop your doctor and ask for a definition or description when your doctor uses a concept or term you do not understand? Advance preparation and orientation for your appointments and meetings with providers, discussed in the next chapter, are critical to avoiding this problem.

In addition, in a recent review, *Consumer Reports'* chief medical advisor suggests that many physicians deliberately use highly technical language in order to control communication and limit patients' questions. Such behavior occurs twice as often when doctors are under time pressure! They seem to speak as if every patient should be able to understand all that they say and all the terminology used.

The following communication strategies — not always practiced! — could help:

- Categorizing
- Signposting
- Summarizing
- Repeating
- Clarifying

- Using simple models and diagrams
- Asking patients to repeat in their own words the information they've just been given

Patient-provider "disconnect." What type of information do patients and providers want most? Based on my experience, patients place the highest value on information about diagnosis, causation, and prognosis for their condition (although they may not know how to clearly communicate this).

> "Do your providers understand the stress levels that you suffer from, and that every appointment is a possible oasis of hope?"

However, because of doctors' traditional emphasis on the injury — and not on the overall experience caused by it — providers may misinterpret your desire for information concerning treatment and therapies to be merely a desire to "just take the pain away."

According to patient reports, in an interview lasting twenty minutes, providers may average little more than *one minute* on the task of giving information. Doctors in general practice overestimate the time they spend in explanation and planning. Simultaneously, they underestimate their time spent discussing the risks of medication, your ability to follow the treatment plan, and your opinion about prescribed medication.

Patient memory. Do your providers understand the stress levels that you suffer from your chronic pain? Do they realize that every appointment is a possible oasis of hope for further relief? Do you and your providers assess just how present and focused you are for each encounter? Do you both understand how often something said — or unsaid — in a meeting can send you into an emotional tizzy?

All of these stress and emotional responses can affect what you take away from your encounters. In fact, it is common for patients to be unable to recall all that their doctor said in a meeting, or to be unable to make sense of difficult messages. On average, patients recall only 50 to 60 percent of the information given by their doctors. Even if you're able to remember more than that, you may not always understand the meaning of key messages, or you might understand in the moment but not necessarily be committed to your doctor's perspective, which will also affect your ability to remember what was said.

Lack of empathy and understanding. With any kind of medical or supportive intervention, but even more so with interventions for chronic pain, a solid relationship based on mutual feelings of trust, respect, and rapport is central to recovery. However, sometimes, despite your own — and your provider's — best attempts, this quality of relating does not happen.

A strong and trusting relationship between patient and provider is absolutely necessary for optimal success in treatment. It may be hard to acknowledge how dependent you are on your providers — not just to treat you but for you to feel well cared for and cared about — but it's true.

Creating strong relationships is a skill not everyone has developed, whether patient or provider. One certainly cannot assume that all doctors, during their medical training, acquire the ability to communicate empathically with their patients. This despite the fact that studies have shown a physician's level of warmth and friendliness to be one of the most important variables in patient satisfaction and compliance. Both physicians and patients may be poorly attuned to their own nonverbal communication: eye contact, posture, nods, distance, and communication of emotion through face and voice.

You may see your doctor as your superhero, there to rescue you from suffering and vulnerability. Your doctor, however, may not understand that, in your chronic pain, you need to experience their connection and caring. If your provider is not respectful or capable of this, much of their and your work may be undermined. It will be harder for you to benefit from their expertise, and harder for you to take responsibility for complying with their instructions. Many people in chronic pain have told me that they see their providers as lacking empathy and respect, and having limited interest or understanding of them as a unique persons.

Do your current providers seem to care about what matters to you in your treatment? Do they seem respectful if you disagree with their recommendations, or have trouble complying with treatment? A large percentage of the people with chronic pain that I have worked with feel that their complaints and concerns were not asked about, and that any disagreements on the fundamentals of their primary problem weren't treated with respect.

Patients don't always perceive that they and their doctor have found common ground, especially in the decision-making process, which should involve a mutual discussion of treatment options and goals and roles in management and should include getting feedback. Adding to this problem is one typical fear: that if you challenge or disagree with your providers, you will get "fired."

Meetings with your providers are likely to become dysfunctional if there are mutual shortcomings in communication. It's important for you and your providers to specifically address the particular reason for your attendance at each visit. This reason will vary over time. Be prepared to clarify your needs to your providers on each occasion. The clearer you are, the less likely you are to experience a communication breakdown.

Legal concerns. In addition to the above list of common patient-provider communication problems, there are legal aspects of poor medical communication to consider. It is part of your legal right as a patient to have the optimal level of effective communications from your providers about all aspects of your care. Be aware that your providers may not be mindful enough about the frequency and importance of communication breakdowns between you. While you can pursue legal action if providers' communication and attitudes are inadequate, your communication with them is more likely to improve if you can be candid and assertive about any issues you encounter. So be on the lookout for the following problems in communication:

- You feel neglected or deserted by your provider.
- You feel information is delivered poorly.
- You feel your provider fails to understand your perspective.
- You feel your views are not valued.

Incorrect Beliefs, Assumptions, and Expectations

The communication issues described in the previous section include those that both parties bring to the provider-patient relationship. In addition, our beliefs and expectations color our perception of events. Expectations, assumptions, and beliefs you and your provider hold can determine both actions and reactions in treatment encounters.

Having shared beliefs and expectations with your providers can be a major help in recovery. When they are not shared, and when the differences between your assumptions and expectations and your provider's aren't discussed and compared, it can cause all kinds of confusion, misunderstanding, and disappointment, as well as undermine the basic trust in and quality of the relationship. If you and your providers are unaware that your beliefs and expectations are out of alignment, you may even inadvertently become more vulnerable to seeing yourself as unable to recover and heading toward disability.

A strong alliance between patient and provider is essential to any optimal medical outcome, but it's even more important with chronic conditions that require treatment over long periods of time and that don't always achieve the full extent of the most desired outcome — in this case, complete eradication of pain.

During my initial assessment and meetings with clients, I explore their assumptions, beliefs, and expectations about their condition and discuss what is realistic to expect from treatment. I look to see what they have learned so far about their pain, how well they understand it and their treatment, and where they stand in relation to their treatment experience thus far. People's assumptions, beliefs, and expectations are often at odds with the reality of the situation, and this disconnect can add significantly to their stress about their pain and its impacts.

I then confer with my clients' medical providers about diagnoses and treatment to elicit information that goes well beyond what I have heard or understood. It's not that providers' reports are necessarily ambiguous, incomplete, indefinite, or contradictory; in fact, many providers I work with are excellent communicators. Nonetheless, people with chronic pain can still be left believing that the information they've received is not completely understandable, useful, or legitimate.

What we tend to expect from a doctor is a clear diagnosis and a concrete, positive treatment plan. We want good communication, clear explanations about the patient and provider roles, and education about our condition — what to do for it and why. Importantly, we want to feel well cared for, in that our suffering and need for relief are seen and understood.

Providers have their own expectations. They expect us to be able to explain, with clarity and consistency, our pain experience, our functioning, and what we want from them. They do not expect or want to hear confusing, inconsistent, or unbelievable presentations of symptoms, or unreasonable demands of treatment.

Nobody wants complexity and confusion. However, if neither patient nor provider articulates their beliefs and expectations about diagnosis and treatment, confusion can follow. And this happens often, because both providers and patients regularly fail to take their beliefs and expectations into account. We blindly expect clarity and certainty regarding what is causing the pain, why it hurts the way it does and where it does, how long it will last, and the method of cure. If the conversation leads to a broad range of possible diagnostic answers, such a range of possibilities can make it seem to the patient like the provider doesn't know what's going on. You don't want contingencies in the information your doctor provides; you want a clearly defined answer and solution.

Unfortunately, there are many medical conditions that do not easily lend themselves to diagnosis or treatment. There is tremendous variability in how much pain, dysfunction, and disability different conditions cause, and finding the best treatment approach involves some patience and trial and error.

> "Patients and providers both often assume they are of the same mind about treatment. Often these assumptions are completely wrong."

Let's take a look at what happens when answers aren't simple, when your provider offers qualified explanations or expresses ambiguity, uncertainty, lack of understanding, or confusion about your diagnosis.

What is it like for you when you hear that? Do you feel a little like a guinea pig? You may wonder how they can tell you it's all right, and recommend treatment, when they don't even know what's wrong.

And what if your provider, with the best of intentions, attempts to offer reassuring statements about treatment recommendations? If the recommendations are not well described, or are not connected to the described problem, do you experience reassurance — or confusion, loss of confidence? If your PCP refers you to other providers or specialists, do you take that as a statement of uncertainty — that they have failed to understand or treat your condition? Suppose the specialist is at odds with your referring provider's diagnosis and treatment and offers something quite different, once again failing to meet your expectations, beliefs, and assumptions. When this happens, and when you don't understand that communication is the issue, you may shop for another doctor, which often compounds the problem. (Remember that, given all the types of communication breakdowns discussed previously, neither you nor your provider are likely assessing or discussing the full extent of the impacts of your pain. This alone is often enough to undermine the working relationship between you and your providers and sabotage your treatment.)

In short, patients and providers both often assume they are of the same mind about treatment. They assume they know what the other believes

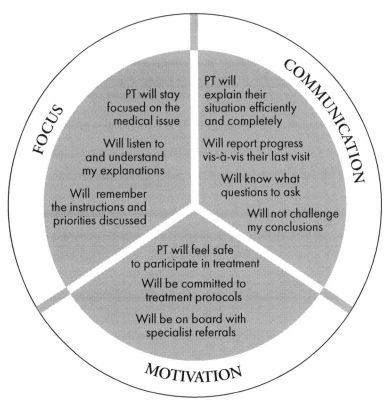

Figure 2. Provider Expectations

and that they have consensus. Often these assumptions, summarized in figures 2 and 3, are completely wrong.

Let me illustrate. I had a client whose doctor said that he was pleased when a follow-up MRI showed no changes in the degenerative disc condition. From the doctor's point of view, "no change" was a positive thing. But my client's reaction to this was silent outrage and deepening depression. She heard "no change" as something negative, and she reacted to the news as if it were a life sentence. Worse still, she did not communicate her reaction to her doctor. She was afraid to challenge his exuberance and authority. (People dealing with chronic pain are often afraid of being labeled as "difficult" by their doctors. They may even be afraid that their needs as patients may contribute to provider burnout.)

When she said nothing, the doctor assumed that she shared his positivity. But my client decided her doctor was insensitive to her needs and sought a new doctor. Had she felt comfortable enough to speak up — or

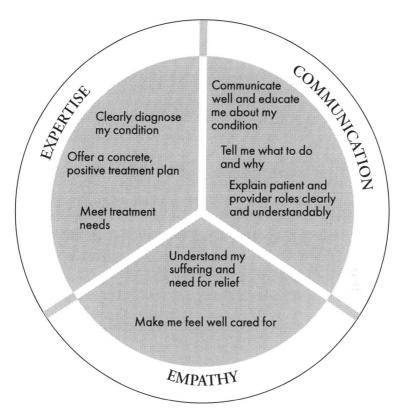

Figure 3. Patient Expectations

had the doctor encouraged her to do so — then this misunderstanding, and its subsequent consequences, could have been avoided.

Another powerful example of the impact of unshared assumptions is seen in the case of Isabella, a forty-five-year-old woman who was scheduled for fusion surgery for her back pain. She believed that there was a high probability she might die or be paralyzed by the surgery. She did not question her doctor about this belief. She assumed the doctor knew she had these fears. Isabella also had a phobia of hospitals because of past negative experiences, and she didn't share this with her doctor either. She assumed he wouldn't understand or have an alternative, and that he'd think she was being difficult.

As a result of her unexpressed fears, Isabella experienced full-blown panic attacks daily for weeks prior to the surgery. This state of mind caused loss of sleep and appetite, along with irritability. She also suffered extreme nervousness on the day of the surgery and during recovery.

Isabella failed to tell her surgeon about her beliefs and fears because she thought he would see her anxiety as needless and unjustified. She herself believed her fears were shameful, and that if the surgeon knew, he'd consider her a "wimp." Because Isabella did not give voice to her worries, the doctor assumed Isabella was in an informed and positive state of mind prior to surgery. This communication breakdown led to serious problems during surgery, and afterward her recovery was undermined to the extent that she needed additional surgery.

Unarticulated and untested provider and patient beliefs, assumptions, and expectations; differences in knowledge, education, culture, experience, personality, personal history, and roles; and different conceptualizations and problems in comprehension — all of this can undo the possibility of finding common understanding. Without this understanding, the likely outcomes will be misinformation, miscommunication, and mutual mistrust. Without this understanding, either patient or provider may reach conclusions that are conflicting, completely off-base, and treatment defeating.

On the face of it, patients' and providers' beliefs and expectations about what they'll receive from each other seem logical and reasonable. However, it's common for them to fail to consider the complexities of human interaction and the problems created by the nature of the treatment environment, and to not consider the role of individual differences in communication and coping skills. Patients often do not comprehend the complexities of the situation, and providers often do not understand the a patient's subjective experience, the extent of their suffering and need for reassurance, and the profound impact chronic pain has produced in their life.

Burdensome Documentation

Documentation demands on providers is another element that may interfere with you getting what you need in treatment. This section is intended to underscore how important it is to make the most of the time you have with your providers, given the other demands on them.

In the treatment environment, paperwork and treatment documentation can take up as much as one-third of a provider's workday. These administrative tasks have become increasingly demanding and hard to accomplish; they are a source of deteriorating professional morale and give doctors less time to get to know you and your pain story. Providers are also doing more medicine with the computer, which does nothing to foster the relationship with their patients.

These demands can also increase the number of errors made. Providers are making clinical decisions with less time to investigate the complexities of your symptoms and with possibly inadequate information obtained from your one-on-one interview. In addition, outside the appointment, they have little time to review your history, drug interactions, contraindications, or the best tests to order for you.

While electronic medical records have increased efficiency by allowing providers to access all of a patient's previous documents, they have also spawned a whole host of electronic ways of bypassing actual patient contact

> "Proliferating administrative tasks are leaving doctors with less time to get to know you and your pain story."

when pressed for time. Providers may rely on notes written by other providers instead of talking to you themselves. These other notes may themselves have been pieced together from previous notes — rather than from current interactions with you. Providers' notes may turn into a cut-and-paste collage instead of an accurate and personalized narrative of illness. Important information, like your reaction to a particular treatment, can be lost in the transfer.

Relying mostly on computer notes for information also increases the chances a doctor will choose the wrong therapeutic course of action. As a case in point, the most common cause of rejection of social security disability applications today is the lack of a coherent clinical narrative across treatment. Without a coherent narrative, it's extremely difficult for evaluators to understand the depth and extent of the factors that contribute to someone's disability. The same difficulty is what many professionals in the medical hierarchy face every day.

Insurance Issues

You may already be well aware of ways in which your insurance coverage can cause you additional collateral damage and even obstruct you from obtaining treatment. The health care reimbursement system can be extremely complicated. Knowing something about how it works and where you can intervene effectively can help you maintain some continuity of care.

Among the potential pitfalls: The rules governing private health care reimbursement change frequently. There are many health care reimbursement plans, and contracts with individual practices and health systems are periodically renegotiated in ways that can affect your costs and your access to care. Providers you need may be in or out of your network, making access to care even more difficult.

In addition, most providers, in order to be in a network, accept a contract rate lower than their billed service. This arrangement may discourage some providers from accepting your insurance. Knowing the payment rules can help you avoid compromises in your access to care. Knowing the extent of the services you need for a holistic treatment approach to chronic pain can help you choose the best option.

Our current insurance system also offers challenges to the number of visits and amount of time you can spend with your providers. The information your primary care or referring provider uses to assess your treatment needs can determine or influence the type and number of visits that will be authorized by your insurance provider, and even whether those visits will be covered at all. The traditional medical approach to pain management may inadvertently fail to request or justify needed treatment.

> "Certain interventions, even if not covered by insurance, are extremely important to your recovery."

Insurance companies, of course, follow the traditional medical approach as well. They do not customarily pay for physical re-activation and post-rehabilitation physical conditioning programs, for instance. They don't cover nutritional planning or psychoeducational classes for pain management. All these interventions are a part of an existential, holistic approach and critically important in people returning to higher levels of functioning. Be aware of these shortfalls in insurance approval: There are certain interventions that, even if not covered by insurance, are extremely important to your recovery.

Treatment Errors

There are many moments in the treatment experience where errors can occur. Some arise simply through the complexity of dealing with chronic pain. Some can unintentionally be brought upon yourself. Over time, the challenge of finding pain relief becomes a powerful, emotion-driven process.

First, identifying a pain treatment that works for you will involve a lot more trial and error than you might expect. In chronic pain, not just the tests but most all of the treatment to some extent are diagnostic and experimental—an effort to narrow down variables and gather pertinent information. It's a necessary approach, but it's also important that you understand the possible negative consequences.

Have your providers clearly explained to you the experimental nature of what they are doing? If these experiments are based on inadequate information about your pain, you may be undertaking unnecessary tests and possibly interventions that make your problem worse, such as unnecessary surgery. Or you may be being undertreated rather than overtreated.

Also, any treatment carries the potential for side effects or complications. For instance, with opioids, you can ask: Will this ease my pain at the expense of my ability to function? Will the treatment mask my real pain generator, or cover over an underlying depression? It's important that you discuss not just pain reduction but the total impact of treatment, including how it may affect preexisting conditions or injuries as well as current medications.

Many people do not understand the structural reason for their pain, so they think they need to keep searching for a magic cure, or at least a reliable diagnosis. These people often pressure their providers for unnecessary imaging tests and surgeries — surgeries that often don't do much to ease their discomfort, but often compound it. As we discussed earlier, mistaken or incorrect expectations probably play a big role in this as well. Meanwhile, time incentives arising from insurance and documentation systems encourage doctors to order imaging tests: It takes longer to sit and reassure someone that their pain will likely resolve on its own than it does to order an MRI.

Other types of treatment errors may occur if providers are not keeping up with and following practice guidelines and recommendations, such as from the American Pain Society and American College of Physicians. For example, data from patients treated for back problems from 1999 through 2010 show an increase in referrals for unnecessary operations and an increase in prescriptions being written for addictive narcotics to reduce pain. At the same time, fewer patients were getting over-the-counter pain relievers such as ibuprofen or acetaminophen, which the guidelines actually recommend as a first-line treatment. Ideally, providers should be aware of and follow approaches that are based on studies showing which treatments work best.

Here are some of the most common treatment errors in chronic pain:

Failing to correctly categorize pain by its cause. Providers sometimes neglect to ask the right questions or perform the proper physical exam when a patient seems to have pain not easily connected to a structural issue. This is called "nonspecific pain," as compared to pain that's caused by a specific structural issue, such as the narrowing of the spinal canal called spinal stenosis, or pain from an acute specific cause such as a fracture. It is still important to determine the elements that contribute to nonspecific pain.

Ordering an imaging test to make a diagnosis. If a patient doesn't have any red flags, providers shouldn't immediately order an MRI, CT scan, or other test to determine the cause of pain. Such tests are warranted only when the physical exam points to a serious underlying condition, and only if surgery or other invasive treatments may be options to treat that condition.

Blaming the pain on the "usual suspects." This error stems from ordering too many imaging tests for hard-to-explain back pain. Often, these tests reveal disk problems, which are then assumed to be the pain generator, but may not be. Studies have shown that most people develop abnormalities in their spinal disks as they age — often without creating pain or being the source of their pain problem.

Forgetting to tell the patient that some pain will resolve regardless of how it is treated. It's important for people to understand that for many chronic pain conditions, there is no quick fix. The body often needs time to heal, whatever injury or muscle strain triggered it.

Overprescribing narcotics and other medications. Medical guidelines say narcotic drugs should be used judiciously and only for people with acute or chronic pain whose pain is severe, disabling, and not controlled with other medications. Narcotics cause substantial risk of drug abuse and addiction. Guidelines also note that chronic use of anti-inflammatory drugs can increase the risk of ulcers and gastrointestinal bleeding.

Underemphasizing and neglecting to refer patients for complementary and alternative approaches. There are many useful alternative approaches to treating chronic pain that have less negative impact upon functioning than traditional medical approaches such as surgery and medication. These include physical therapy, acupuncture, massage therapy, supervised exercise programs, and chronic pain management.

Not understanding the complexity and complications in chronic pain. As you've already learned, there is a great deal that contributes to pain generation, and it's important that you and your providers are attending to all the impacts of chronic pain.

Relying on poor information. Each detail of your pain experience is relevant and important.

Employing a treatment plan that is uncoordinated, unintegrated, and non-comprehensive. This makes it more likely that the premises for making medical decisions will be incomplete or incorrect, leading to more errors.

NEGATIVE CONSEQUENCES OF THE TREATMENT ENVIRONMENT

All of the issues discussed in this chapter can create additional damage in your life, above and beyond your pain. In summary, these are the common negative consequences of the treatment environment:

- Diagnoses that seem ambiguous, indefinite, confusing, and/or contradictory
- Treatment failures with no clear understanding by you or your provider as to why
- Decentralized organization, integration, or management of your treatment, across all providers
- Inadequate time with your providers, compounding confusion about your condition and what to do about it
- Referrals from specialist to specialist in a manner that further compounds confusion or negatively impacts a coherent narrative
- Treatment that creates dependence and disability, such as opioid dependence or provider dependence
- You remaining poorly educated about your condition
- You and your providers lacking a common conceptual model or shared understanding of either diagnosis or treatment
- Side effects or incorrect treatment, which can exacerbate your pain and/or add new physical problems or complications
- Loss of trust in your providers

Subjectively, any of these consequences can leave you not knowing the following things:

- Why you are in pain
- What your provider needs to know about your pain
- What treatments are for or they treatment work or don't work

- What your condition has been diagnosed as and why
- What to do to help your condition within a coherent, comprehensive, integrated treatment plan
- Who is overseeing your treatment
- If you have found the right provider
- If you and your providers have shared concepts about your problem
- Why providers cannot tell you what is going to happen next
- What the most important questions are that you or your providers need to ask, and what information is critical for you and your providers to know
- How much of your life history your providers need to know to understand your needs
- How much to tell your providers about how you feel about their treatment
- Who to trust
- What to expect
- If anyone understands or cares about your suffering and need for relief

So many critical questions can be left unanswered about your condition, your treatment, and your therapeutic relationship with your providers that it can make you particularly vulnerable to the formation of negative pain beliefs (discussed in chapter 15, "Operating-System Impacts"). Negative pain beliefs can affect your life in many ways, including the following:

- Feeling hopeless, powerless, and discouraged about managing your pain
- Feeling discouraged in your efforts at treatment and recovery
- Being fearful of pain, pain exacerbation, and reinjury
- Believing treatment cannot be productive
- Feeling guilty over not recovering
- Believing you are in pain because you are being punished unfairly
- Feeling alone in your suffering
- Believing you are weak and shamed
- Believing you will be stigmatized or marginalized because of your pain
- Believing your pain is permanent
- Feeling fearful of your mortality

When all of the above is taken into consideration, we see how the treatment experience can, rather than alleviate your suffering, substantially add to it. Rather than powering recovery, treatment without sufficient understanding can create fear, confusion, distrust, greater reluctance to engage with the health care system, and a deepening belief that you and your providers are powerless.

In short, such treatment experiences may *enable disability*.

However, finally, there's good news: The next chapter will show you how to take a proactive lead in your treatment situations and empower you to be a full participant in your own recovery.

Chapter 18

Mastering the Treatment Experience

In my study of martial arts, the aim is *mastery*, or deep understanding, of the practice. As students, we know that mastery can only be achieved gradually, over time. Mastering the treatment experience is a bit like that: It takes place within a big system, it takes time to understand it, and progress is best made by small steps and consistent practice.

This entire chapter is devoted to exploring solutions to the inadequacies and breakdowns in communication, failures in planning, and toxic encounters in treatment environments that were described in chapter 17. In presenting these recovery strategies, I outline numerous effective techniques to draw from, and approaches to take to help prevent, address, or overcome the potential problems, obstacles, and damages related to the treatment experience.

Over the past twenty years, and after working with several thousand clients, I have been shocked to find how often it is that people don't understand their diagnosis, treatments, or prognosis. In my intake process, these clients answered self-inventories in ways that indicated, not surprisingly, a high level of dissatisfaction. The anxiety, fear, and frustration reflected in these inventories was profound, and it existed regardless of the competence of any specific provider or that person's substantial and dedicated efforts to treat and care for their patients.

I recommend doing your own self-inventory with the materials in this book's appendixes. This experience is important to a successful treatment plan. Assessing your own level of understanding will help you identify problems you have already encountered or might encounter in the future.

Going through the self-inventory process will also help you orient toward what is essential for a successful therapeutic relationship with your providers and for successful treatment outcomes.

I can't overstate how much a lack of understanding about your condition and treatment path can undermine your treatment and recovery, and, conversely, how much a deep understanding can help ensure the best possible outcome. Remember: Your health care team works for you. They are your providers and consultants and the experts in their fields. But *you* are the expert on your needs and experience. What follows are methods and means to help maximize your chances of a positive treatment experience.

BUILDING A POSITIVE TREATMENT ENVIRONMENT

A treatment environment that is positive and familiar to the whole team can make a profound difference. This is foundational to a successful recovery. Embracing questions, choices, and communications with a sense of confidence and a clear aim will serve both patient and provider and probably even the greater health care system, including insurance providers and the institutions they deal with.

It is a fact that the health care industry is in constant flux, always adjusting to medical advancements, political environments, and economic ups and downs. However, there is much that can be done by patient and provider to create a positive treatment environment. These are some characteristics of such an environment:

- Timely appointments
- Well-informed providers
- A clear and helpful trail of documentation
- Communication that is timely and comprehensible
- Clear boundaries and roles
- Good access to information
- An effective referral system
- A sense of teamwork

Because of the complexity in the treatment of chronic pain, your own initiative and participation in helping to create a positive treatment environment is essential. With the right goals, the right tools, and the right self-knowledge, the investment of time and thought will not prove as daunting as it might first seem. If you are clear about your needs and expectations, if you do your homework and come prepared, and if you engage in a spirit of cooperation and positivity, you will find that it is not that difficult to do.

Willing participation on the part of your provider is of course equally important. I've found most are eager to provide effective and caring services.

This chapter summarizes the intentions, tools, and tips that I have found can best prepare you and your health care team for a positive treatment experience and outcome.

FORGE A PARTNERSHIP

The first step to forging partnerships with your health care providers is to share what your intentions are. And for *you* to know what your intentions are, you must begin with self-knowledge. As you become an aware, educated manager of your pain treatment experience, you will be better able to aid your providers in eliminating or minimizing errors.

> "A positive treatment environment begins with seeing what is and working with what you've got."

The qualities of a good partnership include:

- Mutual respect for each other's needs and roles
- Willingness to be proactive
- Respect for one another's time
- An understanding of one another's pressures
- Skill in communicating efficiently
- Mutual preparedness

In essence, if you and your providers embrace each other's roles as partners in your care, almost all of the potential problems in treatment we explored in chapter 17 can be minimized or eliminated.

A positive treatment environment doesn't happen overnight. Begin with a few steps and remind yourself often that it's a work in progress. It begins with *seeing what is* and *working with what you've got*.

KNOW YOUR INSURANCE

By building a positive treatment environment and being willing to assert your needs and enlist your provider's help, you can also help reduce or eliminate insurance-related issues. It is part of your job to become knowledgeable and informed about necessary documentation for approvals and interventions, to overcome other insurance issues.

But you don't have to go it alone in this task. I have worked with a number of providers who go out of their way for patients who ask for their help with understanding and working with insurance providers. I've known many who are particularly good at advocating for their patients with insurance companies, especially in helping to justify medically necessary treatments the insurance company may initially decline to authorize. The insurance companies themselves can be very helpful in explaining what your policy covers and what is required of you. For those of you sixty-five years and older, seminars and programs exist whose sole purpose is to help educate and assist people in moving their health insurance over to Medicare.

> **"Start thinking of yourself as the quarterback of your health care."**

Paying attention to the important details of your situation can prevent unnecessary documentation. You know the totality of your pain experience, and with good teamwork with your medical providers, your self-knowledge will make a big difference in what is documented and what insurance will pay for. The documentation you can provide includes such things as pain journals, other formal tracking analytics on the impact of pain on your function over time, information on flare-up patterns and management, and other self-reports on the efficacy of treatment. As dry and complex as it may seem, insurance is a fact of modern life, and the more you can bring in terms of accurate information and documentation, the easier it will be to get through the steps.

BE THE QUARTERBACK

To borrow a sports metaphor, start thinking of yourself as the quarterback of your health care. You rely on the expertise of your providers, but you are the one who strategizes the plan and calls the shots. You have a whole team, but you are the strategist when it comes to treating and managing the impact that chronic pain has in your life.

Errors flourish in a climate of ignorance, so let your enhanced awareness of your own chronic pain experience shine a light on your treatment plan and interactions. The more you are empowered in your role in treatment, the more you come to realize that ultimately you need to call the shots as they relate to your recovery. This is the best approach you will have to thriving.

Be holistic in your understanding of how chronic pain affects you and stay focused on the big picture! If you help educate yourself — and your providers where needed — as you progress through treatment, your outcomes will be optimal.

DEEPENING YOUR SELF-KNOWLEDGE

Chronic pain eats up energy, making it easy to skip from day to day along the surface of your experience. But self-knowledge is potent. It has the power to focus your life, to set the tenor of the conversations behind decisions, and to turn despair to inspiration and meaning. Self-knowledge, more than anything else, can change your experience, and this where the

> "Self-knowledge, more than anything else, can change your experience.

concept of mastery comes in: Only you can step into the process of cultivating your own self-awareness. Here are a few strategies to start with.

Pre-Assess Your Experience with Chronic Pain

When someone makes an appointment to see me at my practice, I ask them to fill out a sixty-five-page intake assessment of their pain experience, which includes all relevant personal history and all the impacts they have suffered as a result of their chronic pain condition. This assessment includes:

- Injury history and diagnosis
- Pain experience, physical pain impact, and functional impairment
- History of athleticism and of previous injury
- Medical history, tests, procedures, providers, and treatment history
- Current treatments, treatment experience, personal history, occupational history, and risk factors
- Relationship and family history, relationship assessment, and significant-other impact assessment
- Stress assessment, pain-beliefs assessment, and emotional-impact assessments
- Assessments of impacts on self-regard, self-efficacy, values, coping, and negative belief systems; impact of the event (PTSD); and overall personal impact

I developed this assessment packet over twenty years of client interactions and testimony as to what can happen to someone with chronic pain. Having this information not only informs me about *all* the targets of treatment — thinking it through informs you as well. After filling out my intake packet, most of my clients say they feel that it is the first time anyone has understood what they are going through.

If you had a similar amount of information to give to your providers at the start of treatment, your treatment might proceed in a much more successful manner. Most providers don't ask for or require this level of information from you. But providing it can significantly improve your communication with each other.

> **"Pay more attention to functional impact and less to symptoms."**

With my assessments (some of which — though not all! — are included in the appendixes to this book), I have developed a major aid to your communicating with your providers, setting realistic beliefs and expectations, and ensuring that everyone on your team understands the total impact of your pain.

Know Your Tools for Self-Assessment

As you progress through treatment, continually assess your level of physical vulnerability and your risk of reinjury. There are several tools, listed below, that can help you do this, and achieve self-awareness in other ways as well.

The cure-versus-recovery distinction. Understand the difference between treatments designed to cure, treatments expected to be temporary, and treatments that are rehabilitative.

The pain-versus-injury distinction. Understand that there is a distinction between your pain and your injury. This topic is covered in depth in chapters 4–10 (part 2) on the physical experience .

The function-versus-symptoms distinction. Pay more attention to your functional impacts and less to your symptoms. For example, knowing the symptoms of depression is not nearly as important as knowing how those symptoms affect your day-to-day life. A good description of your functional experience is often more critical information — for both you and your providers — than a description of your pain experience. It's less helpful to say "I get a throbbing headache every morning" than to say "The throbbing headache I get every morning prevents me from starting work on time, is damaging my relationships with my kids, and scares me — that it will always be this way." (That said, accurate descriptions of pain itself do have important implications.)

The language of pain. Understand the diagnostic value of pain-quality descriptions. These are found in your own descriptions of pain. My time and experience with clients have revealed consistent correlations between someone's descriptions and actual structural issues. For example, *sharp* tends to be muscle-related; *achy*, *sore*, and *dull* often signal structural inflammation; *burning*, *shooting*, while *electric shock* typically describes nerve-related pain. Each kind of pain experience relates to a specific structural aspect of your body, and each treatment targets one or more of these structural aspects. Knowing which treatment is for which aspect will help to diminish the mystery of these interventions.

> "Track information about your experience and your treatments. This helps you begin to see patterns."

Tracking records. Create systems for tracking the impact of treatments. Remember: Treatment is not just curative, but also diagnostic. Your system can be simple, such as a small notebook you keep in your pocket, or more elaborate, such as a spreadsheet, but it should record what treatments were undertaken when, who prescribed or administered the treatment, and what changes, if any, you noticed.

Journals. Record in a journal the impact of your treatments, distinguishing between impact on overall function (range of motion, activity level, other functioning) and impact on pain (aching, throbbing, and so forth). Track dates, time of day, observations, notes about what helps and what doesn't, and context (where you were, major events of the day). All of this information can help you begin to see patterns and to accurately answer questions from providers such as "When did this start?" or "What helped the most?"

Flare-up plans. With the aid of your providers and through ongoing assessment of what helps when your pain flares, develop a physical flare-up plan. For example, your plan may be to take medication, lie down, meditate, and later stretch and exercise. You may need to learn to pay attention to the pattern of what can give you relief, or experiment with various combinations. Be sure to ask yourself to understand the meaning to you of your flare-up. Plan for the emotional flare-up that usually accompanies a pain flare-up, such as increased anxiety, anger, and depression. Be aware that you may experience pain flare-ups as traumatic, if they have happened often enough.

Assessment forms. Use any assessment forms you have access to to track your progress in treatment and document variables that may influence treatment outcomes. For example, you may want to document the role that physical de-activation, drug interactions, or psychosocial stressors may have played in your pain. Appendixes A and B offer a few assessment forms that you can copy and use repeatedly over time (or download from newoptionsinc.com) to track what has changed in your experience. You can also find a number of self-assessment tools on the internet. What is most important is to cover all the dimensions of your pain experience as discussed in this book, holistically and across time, and so the assessments can reveal useful patterns in your experience that can aid in recovery. Look for assessments with formats that take advantage of modern analytics and that easily generate user-friendly spreadsheets, charts, and graphs.

> "Knowing yourself means recognizing your gut feelings, reflecting on your behaviors, and being honest with yourself about your situation."

Structural-change assessments. Understand and self-assess any structural impact of treatment that you can observe, such as reduced inflammation, increased muscle cramps or contractions, or a change in numbness or tingling.

Enhancers assessments. Assess the things that enhance treatment for you, such as diet, exercise, meditation, treatment combinations, or spending time with friends and family.

Examine What You Bring to the Table

Knowing yourself means recognizing your gut feelings, reflecting on your behaviors, and being honest with yourself about your situation. What you believe and what assumptions you hold form the foundation of your expectations, and should be identified as part of your treatment plan.

With my clients, I make a comprehensive assessment of their assumptions, beliefs, and expectations. This assessment is intended to provide structure for our decision-making and a framework for getting needs met. As such, it is a useful tool for adaptation and recovery. Many beliefs and assumptions serve well-being, such as believing that putting your hand in a flame will injure you, or assuming that breaking the law will have negative consequences. They are based on experience or common facts and become part of a general way of operating that, in most cases, promotes survival and flourishing. But basing beliefs on speculation, supposition, incomplete facts, predispositions and biases, or fear will not promote flourishing. Instead, it is more likely to undermine your safety and compromise your survival.

Unfortunately, holding false beliefs and assumptions also happens to be a convenient method of oversimplifying the complexities and realities of life. This is frequently the case in the treatment of chronic pain. A person may believe that providers can understand every condition, that every injury has a cure, and that every condition can be successfully treated — when this is not always the case. They may very well want to believe their providers automatically know how to read them and interpret their words, know all about their injury, and know exactly what to do to help.

You, too, may assume your providers know what elements of your pain experience you most want help with. Is your priority to reduce pain sensation? To restore functioning? To understand your physiology? What do you expect when you walk into your provider's office?

Expectations in and of treatment should be based on the reality of your entire situation. This is critical to anticipating and planning for success in recovery. When you base your expectations on false premises, it will more than likely create more stress and disappointment and a lower likelihood of thriving.

So, when strategizing for chronic pain treatment, base your assumptions and beliefs upon facts. These facts may be obtained in the following ways:

- Achieve an understanding of what to look for in your treatment experience, and where your assumptions and beliefs can interfere.
- Develop an awareness of the most relevant information you will need to achieve actual facts about all aspects of your experience.
- Use the samples of the comprehensive holistic-impact assessments from my intake packet (found in the appendixes), or from similar assessments found online.
- Engage in a thorough questioning of your providers, on an ongoing basis, concerning every aspect of diagnosis, treatment, and prognosis, supplemented by your own tracking of your entire experience.
- Do your own guided independent research (as discussed in the next section).
- Collate and compare all feedback from all your providers for consensus and consistency.

When you proceed with this level of engagement, you will construct expectations that are more realistic and better support and empower your recovery.

This is especially true when both you and your providers are aligned in this approach. Without facts, any prediction from a provider (or inside your own head), even if offered with the best of intentions, can be emotionally debilitating and discouraging. Proceed with an open mind. Become an investigator into unchartered territory—which is most likely what chronic pain treatment is for you. Do not assume you and your providers are necessarily on the same page about any aspect of your diagnosis and care, or that you and they define concepts in the same fashion.

The more you understand about your own beliefs, assumptions, and expectations, and consider those of others' as well, the more efficiently you will be able to move through your treatment.

Do Your Own (Guided) Research
Being well informed about your situation saves time. It helps your providers be more successful in their job of delivering treatment. But you will also need guidance as to what you need to know and where to look for information. Ask your providers what they want you to be familiar with about your condition and treatment and if they can recommend good websites where you can read about it. They can be extremely helpful in providing you with appropriate sources of information for accurate and understandable data. Start by taking notes of relevant information at your meetings. And ask your providers to clearly define their expectations about their role and your role—your "job description" as a patient.

> "Ask your providers to clearly define their expectations about their role and your role – your 'job description' as a patient."

Some providers may be reluctant to have you do your own research, but it's unrealistic, especially with modern access to information, to expect you not to do it. It is in your provider's best interest to direct you in this regard, rather than leave it to chance.

Below are several possible avenues and tools for independent research:

The internet. A well-informed consumer makes better choices. Starting with provider-directed internet sites, you can easily locate basic, definitional information about your diagnosis, treatment recommendations, treatment techniques and processes, as well as possible prognoses based upon statistics. If you have just received a diagnosis, a straightforward search term (such as "what's a herniated disc?" or "shoulder anatomy") can lead you to good, basic information that may help you save time in upcoming appointments. You can research statistics on treatment outcomes and even read published scientific research papers on scholar.google.com. You can also search for information about your provider to learn a bit about them and their approach. Your exposure to a broad sampling of material will help you have a more reasoned approach to your expectations about process and outcomes of treatment. It will save time at appointments and allow you to focus on more complicated details of critical importance. It will help you obtain more information from your providers on the deeper aspects of your condition and your providers' experience in dealing with it. It will allow you to make much more informed decisions about your care.

Review the information you have gathered before your meetings with providers so that you are oriented and informed. This will save time on your provider's part in explaining the basics of your condition, and you'll be less anxious and more empowered in the process.

In addition to researching your condition, research techniques for managing chronic pain. Specifically, explore the techniques included in the biopsychosocial model for managing pain. (The biopsychosocial model uses physical, psychological, social, cognitive, emotional, and behavior measures, along with their interactions, to assess a person's pain condition and treat it. It treats pain as a multidimensional dynamic interaction among these factors and explains how they influence one another. These concepts are embedded throughout this book, along with the existential approaches that include the biopsychosocial techniques and go beyond it.)

YouTube. YouTube is a unique source of data. Though it's wise to proceed with caution and never rely on one opinion, YouTube nonetheless offers the opportunity to select the videos that best fit with your learning style and preferences. Information is provided in a variety of ways: diagrams, charts, other media content, and even live patient diagnosis and treatment videos. It allows you to view multiple and varied perspectives on your diagnosis, treatments, and prognosis. You can literally get multiple "consults."

In addition, if you view a number of videos about diagnosis and treatment that are all in accord, it will reassure you that the information your providers are supplying you with is reliable and valid. It will also help you better understand the different perspectives and approaches of specialists. This will significantly reduce your anxiety about understanding your diagnosis and treatment and empower you in embracing your providers' recommendations. Doing this independent learning can lower your fears about what to expect and your frustrations about where you are in the treatment process. It will motivate you to actively comply with your responsibilities in the treatment regimen.

Podcasts. Podcast interviews can be wonderful sources of information, especially if you prefer listening over reading. You can learn about various experts' approaches and patients' experiences in an accessible and conversational style. Using a podcast app, you can subscribe to favorite podcasts on pertinent topics both general (chronic pain, say) and specific (fibromyalgia, for example). Listening to a diversity of opinions can help you learn to be open and discerning and can give you ideas about topics or questions to discuss with your providers.

Your own resource library. Create your own resource library pertaining to your condition — books, articles, links, handouts, and resources organized in a way that's easy for you to access. You can use online bookmarks, physical file cabinets or computer folders, or labeled boxes. On the computer, learn to take screenshots so you can capture charts or pictures. Keep up on research concerning your condition. With the pace of change and development in modern medicine (and everything else), never assume you are fated to rely only on your current treatment options.

Coming to know yourself, your fears and hopes, your motives and expectations, and, literally, your aches and pains is a rewarding undertaking, with benefits beyond good health care. By looking closely at *what is*, you are that much closer to *what could be*.

PREPARING FOR YOUR ENCOUNTERS

Time is at a premium with your providers, and it's important to figure out how best to utilize that time for optimal outcomes.

It's important to arrive at appointments prepared and knowing what you hope to achieve in the time allowed, with your questions ready and your report about your status formulated and organized. The strategies below will help you build this skill set.

Remember: Preparation is a decision you make. It's a commitment to take time before your appointment to prepare your thoughts and time afterward to distill and record what you come away with.

Schedule Ahead

If you have chronic pain, chances are you will have to see your providers multiple times. Like many patients, you typically schedule one appointment at a time. This often creates large gaps in time from one appointment to the next, especially with providers who are in great demand.

I cannot emphasize enough the emotional cost of delays in treatment and their potential to exacerbate the negative physical impacts of your pain. Too much delay can mess up continuity and progress in treatment. This is especially true where there is a break in care for one of the following reasons:

> "Problems with timing occur when neither you nor your providers realize that you are in a state of ongoing crisis."

- Your provider hasn't scheduled you frequently enough.
- Your provider hasn't made a necessary referral.
- Your provider hasn't requested a reauthorization from your insurance company for additional treatment.

If you have to wait too long or aren't able to communicate with your provider about negative developments in your condition, new fears, or new frustrations, it is likely to substantially increase your anxiety and frustration and stress. There is a reason why stress management is at the center of psychological care for chronic pain. Stress has the power to dramatically increase your pain and to suck the energy out of your motivation to recover.

These problems with timing occur when neither you nor your providers realize that you are in a state of ongoing crisis. Time passing matters. Each day of suffering is another day you must struggle to hold onto what is left of your life. This creates existential stress, the most powerful type of stress. Knowing this, you can be proactive in scheduling more frequent appointments.

Do not wait until the day of your appointment to schedule the next one. At the outset of treatment, discuss with your providers a plan of action that covers as many appointments as it's possible to anticipate needing. If you schedule two or three in advance, you'll be able to space them apart at appropriate intervals, and avoid having to go too long between appointments when the provider's calendar fills up.

Prepare Your Questions

Waiting until you are with your providers to remember or think of questions that are important to you can be an unreliable approach. You may be anxious and forget, or you may feel rushed. If you haven't prepared, you may not ask the most relevant, needed, or important questions. Formulating your questions in advance is an important part of preparation.

> "Formulating questions in advance is an important part of preparation."

Here are some examples of important questions to reflect on, research, or have prepared to ask your providers:

- What is the exact anatomical or structural explanation for my pain condition?
- How will activities — or lack of them — affect my pain? (Specify the activities that are important to you.) Do I need to stop these activities, or can I modify them?
- How long am I likely to be in pain?
- What benchmarks might I see? What is the likely course of my recovery?
- Will I eventually be able to resume my regular activities? (Again, specify the activities that are important to you.)
- How is this treatment likely to affect my pain problem? What are the possible side effects?
- What is my ultimate prognosis?
- Why does my structural problem cause the specific pain in each specific area? How does it work as a system to produce pain?
- Are there factors or influences other than my structural issues that contribute to or cause any of my symptoms? (For example, posture, de-activation, de-conditioning, compensation, pain attention, medication, treatment side effects, and any other impacts discussed in this book.)
- Be aware that the answers to the above questions may exceed the time allotted to a single visit with your provider. Prioritize your questions and make a plan to get them all answered over time.

If you are seeing a specialist, focus your questions on their area of specialization — information that they will know and understand based upon their training and experience. A surgeon, for instance, will be able to give you specific information that your primary provider may not, and vice versa.

Develop your list of questions, basing them on what seems logical to you. Then prioritize them, as there may not be time to address them all in one appointment. And, importantly, make sure your questions are relevant to whatever it is that causes you the most anxiety about your diagnosis, treatment, and prognosis.

Send Questions in Advance

Once you have compiled and prioritized your questions, date your list, make a copy for yourself, and send a copy to your provider's office — by mail, fax, or email — so that it arrives four to seven days before your appointment. Request that the list of questions be put in your chart, and that the provider be made aware of your list prior to your visit.

Take your copy of your questions to your appointment. Since you may have more questions than can get addressed in one session, also bring a short agenda of what you hope to accomplish during your time with your provider that day. This will help you and your provider be more focused, and you to be less anxious during your meetings.

This action on your part accomplishes several things. Besides making your questions available to your providers in advance, it also makes them part of your medical legal record. This alerts your future providers as well about what you need to know. But here's the biggest benefit: This action will make the most efficient use of your time with your provider, thus making it more likely that you will get the information you need. It will also help maintain continuity of care. (Continuity of care is an approach concerned with maintaining the quality of health care provided over time. It is a process that includes shared documentation and proper communication between providers when referrals are made.)

If some questions go unanswered during the session, or new questions arise, don't wait for your next appointment to address them. Email or fax these questions to your provider as soon as you can, with a request for feedback as soon as possible. Again, be sure to request that your inquiries be included in your chart.

This process may seem work-intensive. You may be concerned about how your providers will react. It has been my experience that they will appreciate your efforts. If necessary, explain how your questions will help them accomplish their mission in the limited time they have for your meetings and provide more value for you. If you encounter any resistance, ask how they would like to handle your questions and in what other ways your concerns can be addressed.

Take the Composite Approach

Specialization can compound the problems in treatment for people with chronic pain. For many chronic pain conditions, it can be difficult to understand the information about the condition, treatment recommendations, and treatment outcomes from even a single data source, let alone a variety of them. Each of your multiple providers has a common understanding of your condition as well as a unique understanding about what to do about it. Consider, for example, a general practitioner, a physiatrist (rehabilitation specialist), a physical therapist, an acupuncturist, and a surgeon: Their perspectives on understanding the human body, physical systems, and how injuries manifest and need to be treated will all differ according to the lens of their specialty. The *composite approach* involves detailed questioning and note-taking with each of your providers about these two elements:

> "The collective information compiled from multiple providers will often be more informative than any single perspective."

- The specifics of the structural issues that are causing your pain
- How your treatment interventions are designed to address these issues

Use the same questions with each provider and compare their responses, looking for similarities and, especially, agreement. The collective information will often be more informative than the input from any single provider, and you will find that, overall, you can get a more three-dimensional, holistic understanding of what is going on.

Reconceptualize Your Time

It's hard to appreciate just how much information and meaning can be contained in just one minute. Consider the typical TV commercial: One commercial spot is usually only fifteen or thirty seconds long, but subjectively that time can feel like minutes or more. Why? Because it's so engaging — advertisers have learned how to present a wealth of detailed information by giving exquisite attention to the words and images they use, the associations they create, and the way all are intertwined to tell a story. They spend hundreds of thousands of dollars on those few seconds to create a connection, often by association, and to capture our attention and appeal to whatever aspects of being human they can most easily connect to. They know what message they want to send, and what effect and outcome they want to create. They can appeal to our values, shared experiences, intelligence, humanity, compassion, pleasure, sympathy — to anything we value as people or as a society. They understand that human interaction is a creative experience where, to a large extent, we can determine the outcome.

Typical encounters with health care providers are between fifteen and forty-five minutes — the equivalent of 60 to 180 commercials. Do not dismiss the value of that time because you do not believe it is enough. Think about how you can maximize the value of this time — how you can condense your message, how you can connect.

With that in mind, plan your "commercial." What message do you want to give your provider? Do you want to be perceived as someone who complains and can only talk about how much you hurt? More likely, you want to be perceived as being honest and forthright, as someone bringing

> **"Be assertive about all your needs, not just the physical ones."**

your real experience — the totality of what is happening to you — to the table: your physical suffering; the small, day-to-day manifestations of your condition; and your reactions to treatment. You want to be known as the person most in search of recovery.

You are the most qualified person to attest to the damage chronic pain is creating in your life. Go beyond your usual sense of social propriety, if necessary. Do not be overly concerned about being negatively judged for having, at best, mixed feelings about your condition, providers, and treatment. Be assertive about all your needs, not just the physical ones that medical treatment aims at. Your providers need to have information about the life context they are prescribing in and how this unfolds for you as a unique individual.

Cultivate What You Bring to the Table

There are multiple approaches to good communication that involve mobilizing intrapersonal skills such as vulnerability, assertiveness, and the ability to handle conflict. These aspects of communication can play a major role in preventing or countering communication breakdowns. Consider the role each of the following important traits and skills could have in ensuring effective communication:

Vulnerability. You may not appreciate how valuable your vulnerability can be to success in treating your chronic pain. It's often hard for people to acknowledge that they are hurting. It can be even harder to admit they are also afraid, angry, or feeling helpless, hopeless, and clueless. But sharing these thoughts and feelings with others appeals to our common human experience. We all have these thoughts and feelings at times. It seems counterintuitive, but acknowledging them can help create true intimacy.

Think about the greatest human strengths and all the many ways needs can be met. Paradoxically, the most powerful state you can be in is your own vulnerability. Yet it remains a much-maligned state. What is the power of vulnerability?

> "Paradoxically, the most powerful state you can be in is your own vulnerability."

In vulnerability, we find our humanity. It is our highest level of humanness. We all are truly in need of help at times, pressed and limited at various moments in our life, regardless of who we are, what we know, all we have done, and all we will be. When we find ourselves vulnerable, the greater the need, the deeper the vulnerability. Yet we reject vulnerability as a negative, as a weakness, as something to be avoided, not shared.

Vulnerability involves revealing to yourself and others your innermost needs and feelings, without judgment or critique. There are various levels of vulnerability, starting with being truthful with yourself. Through acknowledging the negative realities in your life without judgment, you can move on to expressing your feelings about those negative realities and then dealing with what is driving them. These negative realities can include feelings that many people consider shameful or unacceptable, such as anxiety, anger, sadness, and grief. Be willing to share these feelings, including with your providers. They have these same feelings, just like you, about any kind of suffering they have ever experienced.

Vulnerability is *the* common human denominator. We all have needs and feelings. We have all experienced some form of emotional or physical suffering. By sharing your needs and feelings, you make it possible for others to better connect and understand what you are experiencing and how to relate in helpful ways. It can help to produce a common understanding of what it means to you to have chronic pain. Providers do not have to have experienced chronic pain themselves to understand your emotional suffering. This is also true about confusion and uncertainty. We have all been there. There is no shame in not being able to handle something none of us was trained or prepared for.

If you can be vulnerable with your providers, it will break many of the artificial barriers and breakdowns identified in the section on communication problems in the treatment environment. To do this, you must open yourself to others for reflection and investigation. But you're also opening yourself to receive comfort, support, solace, and, most importantly, connection. There is great power in openness and uncertainty. Understanding what you do not know reveals what you need to know. You may find this difficult, but the results will be rewarding — in what you get in return and how you feel about yourself.

Your feelings about your condition, the state and rate of your recovery, your treatments, and your relationship with your providers are critical data. You may be reluctant to share these feelings with providers, thinking them either inappropriate or intrusive. You may be fearful that the expression of these feelings, especially frustration and anger, will alienate your providers and get you "fired" as a patient. This will not happen if you're skilled at assertiveness and conflict resolution, so read on!

Assertiveness. Chronic pain and the treatment environment around it can challenge the most skilled individual. When medical conditions are hard to diagnose and treat, or when they are incurable, it creates a different emotional climate in treatment encounters and a different mindset for you and your providers. This may be compounded by the fragmentation of your treatment among specialists and any lack of coordination of care.

I have worked closely with many fine providers of many different healing disciplines over the years. They work hard to provide whatever they can to help their patients, but their medical options are limited. This is especially true if they do not embrace a holistic model of care that addresses the psychological, social, and emotional aspects of human needs. The result is that they're often anxious and frustrated that they can't do more for you. They know that their limits impede their mission to heal. Even those who want to help the most often must convey bad or disappointing news.

Many people cannot believe that their providers really understand their suffering and need for relief. Trust me, they do. However, it's harder for providers to connect when they perceive their patients as complaining about and catastrophizing their pain. Also, people with chronic pain — which is to say, people in crisis — frequently react to failed or limited treatment outcomes with anger and frustration, and this may produce similar feelings in their providers. These patients and providers may end up treating each other as enemies, not allies.

> "When you don't understand why you're not getting what you need, be assertive and investigate – don't assume."

If a negative emotional climate builds between you and your providers, it can profoundly undermine your recovery. When people don't get what they want from their providers, they tend to believe that their providers either don't understand their condition or don't care, and trust is lost. A form of dialogue must be created between you and your providers to prevent this.

So, when you don't understand why you're not getting what you need, be assertive and investigate — don't assume. When you are asked by a person in authority to do something that doesn't sound reasonable or doable, ask why you should do it. You need not accept authority without reasonable explanation. Share your experiences as they relate to your providers' recommendations. Do not monopolize the conversation, nor let them monopolize it. Don't be afraid to bring them around to your perspective when it is appropriate and relevant.

It may be helpful here to distinguish between aggressive communication and assertive communication. Communication is aggressive when feelings, thoughts, and needs are expressed at the expense of others. If what you say humiliates, judges, or blames, it will stir up guilt and resentment in the other party. Aggressive communication can contain an air of superiority. It can be cold and deadly quiet or flippant, hard, authoritarian, and loud. Physically, aggression may show in eyes narrowed, glaring, expressionless, or hostile; jaw clenched; gestures that are rigid, abrupt, or intimidating. It may involve pointing fingers or making a fist. It may involve a raised voice and insulting language. In treatment encounters, these behaviors may be interpreted not just as angry and frustrated but as challenging and argumentative.

In effective assertive communication, you make direct, authentic statements regarding your feelings, thoughts, and needs. You represent yourself by standing up for your rights while also respecting the rights and feelings of others. You have the ability to make non-offensive direct requests and direct refusals. You are open and frank about your feelings. In treatment encounters, this approach uses word choice, tone, and body language to communicate your desire to be informative, emotionally honest, and authentic with your providers.

Do not bottle up your emotions, but also do not let your emotions control you. Listen attentively, be empathic, and use negotiation, collaboration, and compromise. Offer constructive feedback without being hostile or defensive. Physically, show your assertive side with a balanced, comfortable emotional posture and a relaxed voice—clear, audible, and firm. If possible, and emotionally comfortable, use direct eye contact without staring; attempt to be at eye level with the person you are speaking to. Your eyes should communicate openness and honesty. Facial expressions should match the feelings you wish to convey (such as smiling to indicate pleasure, serious to indicate anger).

In assertive communication, start by defining the problem specifically ("I think …"). Describe your feelings using "I" messages ("I feel …"); avoid "you" statements ("You don't …"). Avoid making the mistake of disguising one for the other ("I feel you don't …"). Express your requests simply and firmly ("I want …"), and avoid long descriptions and indirect statements. Use short statements and repeat your point without getting sidetracked by irrelevant issues. Offering excuses is not helpful. When you disagree with someone, do not pretend agreement for the sake of "keeping the peace."

Use calm repetition, repeating what you want until the other person gets your point. ("Unfortunately, I don't understand your diagnosis, so could you please explain?") Paraphrase what the other person said, then repeat your point. ("So you're saying that you're unsure as to whether or not treatment will help, is that right?") Ignore the content of someone's anger and try to put off further discussion until they have calmed down. ("I can see that you might have misunderstood my question about treatment. I didn't mean to second-guess your expertise, I was just confused.") Likewise, put off your response to a challenging statement until you are calm

> "If neither you nor your providers are getting what you really want from your encounters, you are primed to be at odds with one another."

and able to deal with it appropriately. ("I would rather talk about that later.") You might offer a workable compromise, or bargain for material goals, but if the end goal involves a matter of self-worth, there can be no compromise. ("I will gladly follow your treatment recommendations if I better understand how they will help.") Don't create a power struggle, but seek collaboration and clarification.

Conflict-resolution skills. It can be quite challenging to find yourself at odds with your providers concerning any element of your care. Your goal is to avoid either alienating the provider or becoming discouraged yourself. However, situations involving chronic pain and treatment are a veritable hotbed for potential conflict. If neither you nor your providers are getting what you really want from your encounters, you are primed to be at odds with one another: Your provider cannot offer to cure you or eliminate your pain, and you cannot get treatment that will totally free you of your suffering. How then is it possible to prevent your encounters from becoming adversarial?

The answer is good conflict-resolution skills. Conflict resolution begins with an understanding of what conflict is. It may seem contradictory, but conflict is the vehicle for building a great relationship. Conflict is not a disagreement or an argument; that's what happens when people don't understand what conflict represents. Understand that conflict is merely a difference. Every conflict is based on a difference in perspective or belief.

A strongly stated difference indicates a person's *commitment* to an idea or choice rather than to the absolute truth. To illustrate, consider people's different political stances on capital punishment — strong beliefs for which people may have great passion and commitment. Yet across all religions, laws, philosophies, and general human opinion, there is no definitive right and wrong. A case can be made for most views.

Likewise, when discussing values, opinions, beliefs, or perspectives about treatment from your providers, there is no absolute truth. Remind yourself that the value in having differences is in the opportunity to find common ground. If someone says or does something that offends or hurts you, before you react, ask yourself: *"Is this a person who would willfully, consciously, or intentionally seek to cause me harm?"* If your answer is no, do not attack — investigate.

In order to investigate, you can use *resolution communication*. These are the four steps to resolution:

1. Ask for permission. If you're concerned the other person will be defensive or hostile when you bring up your differences, inform them that you are perceiving a difference and *ask* if they would be willing to discuss it.

> "If your provider's immediate response is dismissive, then that difference becomes the one to focus on."

2. Give a disclaimer. Disclaim any intent on your part to blame or criticize the other. Admit that the responsibility may fall upon you and that you are prepared to acknowledge this.

3. Give reassurance. Reassure the other that your intent in the discussion is not to prove yourself right. It is to find common ground and to eliminate the negative feeling between you and the other generated by your differences.

4. Pitch your intention. Your pitch is that you are looking to build a positive relationship.

In conflict resolution, be sure to stay focused on the most immediate difference or misattunement. Say you're beginning to have a difference with a provider, such as over what the best treatment approach is. If your provider's immediate response is dismissive, then that difference becomes the one to focus on. Stay focused on the most immediate difference, regardless of what the original mission was. The relationship comes before the individual when there is a difference. Getting needs met in a relationship must be mutual. Conflict resolution is dedicated to mutual satisfaction.

Good judgment, not value judgments. In relationships, value judgments, especially negative ones, can lead to misunderstanding and make it harder to see truth.

Judgmental thinking has several general identifying characteristics. Its statements are absolute and value-based, not fact-based. They are frequently negative, but can be positive. They always accuse, or imply negative character traits or characteristics. They include the stance that being right is all that's important. This kind of thinking occurs when we don't respect differences. When we accept value judgments as truth, we may believe we have the right to impose "the truth" on others and dictate to them what to think and how to feel.

In treatment, you may experience judgment from a provider, or you may be the judgmental one. However, if you can learn to see disagreement as difference and not as rejection, it can help you build a better working relationship. Avoid judging. Seek understanding, cooperation, and consensus.

> "Be respectful of your own emotional state and know that cultivating the quality of your relationship with your providers is part of your recovery."

Self-regard. It may seem contradictory, but to get your needs met when communicating with providers, you need to be effective at self-regard. People often rely on their values, such as "being nice," when deciding whether or not to ask for what they need. This is not the most reliable method for getting your needs met or preventing future conflict. Rather, when your needs conflict with those of a provider's, ask yourself: "If I were being selfish, thinking of what I really need, what would I want to say or do in this situation?"

These are the phases of self-regard:

- Knowing what your needs are
- Understanding that you are entitled to your needs
- Knowing that no person's needs are superior to yours at any moment in time, regardless of your values, and acting accordingly
- Understanding that quality of relationship is what you're seeking

To get the most out of treatment, try to know in each moment exactly what your needs and your wants are. Be respectful of your own emotional state. Act in ways that are true to yourself and make free choices, not ones that can lead to resentment.

Also know that cultivating the quality of your relationship with your providers is part of your recovery. Consider whether the relationship has a good give-and-take. Consider the emotional cost of your choice: Will it get you what you need and strengthen the relationship with your provider? *Then* choose your course of action.

You may be surprised to find that you will act the same way you often have in the past — the main difference being that you will know it was *your choice*, not something imposed by your provider or the treatment environment. Being truly self-regarding in the treatment environment can be the difference between getting what you need or not.

Analysis (of treatment outcomes, side effects, and concerns). You are the subject-matter expert on your pain experience. No one knows how it manifests day to day, moment by moment, better than you. What you know can be vitally important to you, your provider, and your recovery.

> "You are the subject matter expert on your pain experience. No one knows better than you."

To make best use of your information, consider how best to present your information about events over time. In retail sales, for example, you would track daily sales, marketing, and operational matters, and look at data over time to reveal patterns that might help you make improvements and raise your levels of success. Apply this thinking to your condition. Your pain, suffering, and dysfunction are daily events. Knowing them by some daily record is helpful, but tracking them across time will reveal patterns that are much more likely to improve your chances of recovery. More significantly, this approach can reveal what is working or not working in your treatment, the different physical and emotional elements of your recovery, and patterns of flare-ups and setbacks.

For starters, get a copy of your treatment plan and treatment notes. Then keep a written record of all treatment recommendations and outcomes. Try a computer spreadsheet if possible, an efficient way to organize information that you can add to, copy, share, and send. Document your experience in regard to pain reduction, range of motion, range of activity, and level of functioning. Track this between visits using not only daily reports but graphical representations of this information over time. This is the *analytics approach* to pain management. Provide copies of your analyses to providers on a periodic basis to help them understand your progress. This will save a great deal of time and make them far more informed and productive.

Be sure to include a running list of your questions or concerns about the effects of treatment, either negative or positive. By tracking the impacts from treatment over time, you can help your providers better understand what is really happening. This will significantly reduce your anxiety and frustrations about where you stand in the recovery process. It will increase your motivation and commitment to treatment. Never be a blind follower in treatment, just following orders. Question whatever you need to question to enhance your ability to recover.

> "Difficulties arise from the medical environment and the lack of awareness of the existential impact of chronic pain. Both providers and patients suffer from this."

Every step in treatment inspires hopes and fears about your need to be done with suffering. The more that you know about what's happening in treatment and where you stand in your progress, the better. When your treatment is itself painful or traumatic, be sure to document and report all side effects immediately:

- Do not wait for your next appointment.
- Do not "tough it out" or assume it just goes with the territory.
- Do not be concerned about "bothering" your provider.

The timelier your information about treatment impact, the better your provider can manage it. If you're concerned or uncertain about your provider's strategy in your care plan, ask. Do not hesitate to report to your providers any fears, frustrations, or reluctance to follow treatment recommendations. They are the experts on your care plan, but you are the expert on your experience. If they make recommendations that may cause you to suffer, or risk additional injury or exacerbation of your condition, you have a right to ask and a need to know.

INTEGRATING YOUR PROGRESS

The treatment environment is intended to be healing and, in the best cases, curative. Overall, providers are dedicated to helping their patients in any way possible. I have been fortunate to work with many excellent providers over the years. None of them would want any of the difficulties covered in this book to happen. Much of the problem arises from the structure of our medical environment and the lack of awareness of the existential impact of chronic pain. Both providers and patients suffer from this.

Hopefully, the approaches I recommend in this chapter demonstrate that problems in the treatment environment need not be obstacles to recovery. Instead they reveal *possibility* and *opportunity* in the context of what otherwise often appears insurmountable. This is indeed the theme of this entire book. In all the impacts from chronic pain and the problems they create, mastery is both possible and powerful.

Takeaway

An immune system's role is to learn, adapt, and operate in a way that protects the whole. Your existential immune system protects the whole of *you*, and understanding how to support your existential immune system in the complicated context of chronic pain, and other complicated challenges, is key to thriving.

Bottom Line

The benefit of supporting your existential immune system through self-awareness can be simply expressed in this equation:

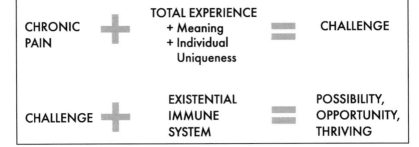

Conclusion

Evolving the Existential Immune System

Conclusion

Two Stories

We now come to the final chapter in this book, whose purpose is to invite you into a full-scale assessment of two of my clients — Ralph and Val — as they presented to me at the beginning and throughout our work together. We will explore how the approach laid out in this book helped them achieve mastery over their pain, going into much more detail than in previous client stories. Now that you have read the rest of this book, you are better oriented to perceiving the complexity of the impacts from chronic pain and understanding how to deal with them. Each story demonstrates the process of analyzing negative realities and using various techniques to optimize potential for recovery.

As already discussed, achieving mastery begins with building awareness of your challenges, the potential of your existential immune system, and its current level of functionality. Most importantly, it begins with understanding that *your ability to adapt and thrive is potentially limitless.*

Ralph's and Val's recovery stories demonstrate both the power of the existential immune system and its adaptability. These individuals demonstrated the high levels of openness to change, curiosity, courage, commitment, hard work, and dedication needed to end a life of suffering and merely surviving and to build a life worth living — even in the context of chronic pain. I hope these stories will demonstrate how respect for individual differences and the diversity of chronic pain problems can be addressed, and illustrate the comprehensiveness, depth, and completeness of the existential approach presented in this book.

RALPH'S STORY: EXISTENTIAL POSSIBILITY

When I first met Ralph, he was suffering from major cervical and lumbar injuries caused by a fall from a ladder at work and experiencing significant pain in many areas of his body simultaneously. "Everything just hurts all the time!" he said, rating his pain at 9 on a 0-to-10 scale. Pain greeted him every morning, "tortured" him during the day, and disrupted his sleep every night. He never woke feeling rested.

Every movement flared his pain: standing, lying down, lifting, coughing, sneezing, changing positions. He experienced his pain as severe, sharp, and stabbing. He believed it was much worse now than when it began, despite several years of many different treatments.

Understanding the Challenge

Ralph had no hope his pain would be better in the future. He had stopped working and stayed home, reclining, or lying down, but with little comfort. It was quite painful for him to get out of a chair or go up a staircase, even with supports. He walked only short distances. His movements were guarded, as any could trigger his pain. Therefore, he constantly had to ask others to do things for him, including all homeowner tasks and chores around the house.

Understandably, Ralph had dropped all his outdoor recreation activities, which had once included traveling, boating, waterskiing, gardening, camping, and hiking. He'd stopped joining family functions or playing with his children. In short, he could not perform any of the roles in his life that mattered to him.

As a lifelong athlete and former marine, Ralph had, prior to his injury, been able to go at tasks with great endurance and drive. He had prided himself on his ability to tolerate pain. But now, 80 percent of his physical conditioning had been lost, in both strength and flexibility. He had gained thirty pounds. Simple actions tired him. He no longer had any of his former physical confidence; his self-image and physical identity were in tatters.

Meanwhile, Ralph's treatment experience was full of problems. With all providers except his most recent, he had experienced confusion and lack of clarity. How much of his experience and needs should he tell his providers about? What information did they need from him? He did not know. And they had not explained his treatments or their plans in ways that Ralph understood. He didn't know what to expect from his treatments—or whether they were even safe. He didn't understand exactly what was causing his pain, how treatments were supposed to help, and which outcomes were realistic. He was fearful of his pain, of flare-ups and reinjury, and of his rehabilitation activities. His greatest fear was that he would be permanently disabled.

Ralph had not felt reassured by his providers, nor guided in how to be safe in his movements. Did his providers understand his needs? Did they really care about his suffering? Ralph believed not. He felt no sense of partnership with them.

Ralph's medications at the time we met — including gabapentin, tizanidine, and oxycodone — were causing more physical and cognitive dysfunction than reducing pain. He also was using alcohol and cigarettes, to the point of addiction, in an attempt to help control his pain.

The impact of all this on Ralph's life, plus his lack of progress in treatment, had led him to some strong disempowering beliefs about his pain. He felt helpless, hopeless, and discouraged to effect any change in his pain condition. In his words, he believed his pain was "horrible, intolerable, impossible to handle or function with." He felt wrongly punished. He thought he must be "a weak person" because he could not handle the pain. He believed his pain problems were too complex and hidden for his doctors to understand, that the pain was permanent, that his life was ruined. He had started to believe that no matter how much he tried, things would just keep getting worse.

Damage to Relationships

At the time of his injury, Ralph was forty-two years old. He'd been married for many years to his high school sweetheart and had two teenage children. After completing high school and some college, he'd worked as a home improvement expert for over twenty years and had been quite satisfied and successful in his career. Now he felt his opportunities fading away.

Before his injury, Ralph and his wife had had a strong, satisfying relationship. Afterward, they experienced more friction, arguments, and building resentments against each other. These began to redefine their relationship, driving them further apart. Both became increasingly anxious, angry, and alienated from each other. Ralph believed his wife was having an affair. And his relationship with his children had begun to unravel as well. Ralph avoided them, physically and emotionally, lest they see his "weakness" and be "disappointed" in him.

From a young age, Ralph had been expected to help care for his younger siblings. He said he had felt "robbed" of his childhood and described his mother as "mean, stubborn, controlling, selfish, and fake." Ralph's dad had been physically abusive. Now Ralph's pain, his experiences in treatment, and his family's reaction to his condition were stirring up these traumatic childhood experiences and evoking PTSD-like symptoms.

Ralph had valued being courageous, honest, responsible, ambitious, self-controlled, and totally self-reliant. He preferred to be stoic, to keep negative feelings to himself. The coping strategies he liked to rely on were common sense, practicality, resourcefulness, and humor. But the sheer weight of the damage to Ralph's life was beyond the capacity of his usual ways of coping, and he was finding it increasingly hard to get what he wanted and needed. Another tough thing was that his self-esteem seemed to be dependent on his productivity and success — which was untenable.

Over time, Ralph's condition included ever-increasing impacts. With marital stress, social isolation, financial worries, and a lack of pleasurable experiences, Ralph felt that he was "dysfunctional, useless, and powerless." Many days, nothing could cheer him up. Each day he felt more anxious, tense, and worried. His whole life felt unsafe. Pain and limitations left him frustrated and angry — all day, every day.

As you can see, Ralph's injuries and their collateral damages had created many negative realities in his life. They had demolished his lifestyle. They had interfered with, and possibly thwarted, all his pursuits and goals. They had reduced his economic status and challenged his ability to be productive in any meaningful way. They had undermined his ability to take good care of himself and provide for his family. They had caused significant damage to his social activities and relationships. Ralph's pain had undermined the possibility that he might enjoy his future life.

Damage to Self

Inside himself, Ralph became increasingly sad and discouraged. He had lost his sense of accomplishment and productivity. He was finding it harder and harder to enjoy people or to feel close, affectionate, or loving. He struggled to feel lighthearted. His self-esteem was crashing, and he was losing a positive sense of himself. He began to feel worthless and struggled to feel any sense of value. Ralph did not feel likable, respectable, lovable, or good about himself.

Nothing he did made him feel calm, relaxed, safe, secure, peaceful, or free of worries. He was beginning to avoid engaging with anything or anyone. He had lost almost any sense of pleasure in life. Once full of the joy of life, Ralph had begun to doubt that life was worth living.

Ralph had lost his sense of well-being. His memory, concentration, attention, and focus all seemed compromised. These troubles interfered with him learning new things or having new and satisfying experiences. His pain experience left him feeling alienated from others. He struggled to cope, unsuccessfully. He felt insecure, unsafe, and ashamed of himself. In short, it was hard for Ralph to believe he could continue to be the person he wanted to be.

Anyone would be overwhelmed by the awareness of so much loss. But paradoxically, this awareness set the stage for Ralph's path to recovery and thriving.

Engaging the Existential Operating System

When we first met, it was quite challenging for Ralph to engage in a trusting relationship with me. This began to change as Ralph filled out the extensive intake packet I use, which highlighted all the dimensions of his extensive collateral damages and of his current existential operating system. When Ralph and I reviewed the findings together, it was enlightening to him — and helped him realize that I actually understood what was happening to him in a comprehensive and meaningful way. He said that for the first time in his journey through treatment, he felt heard and understood. This gave him the courage to consider trusting me and to try to deal more effectively with his pain — a major shift in awareness.

> **"Paradoxically, acute awareness of loss sets the stage for your path to recovery and thriving."**

I suggested that rather than talking about pain and mental health issues, we would focus on defining the existential impact of his pain and the necessary upgrades to his existential operating system.

Ralph had physical problems and persistent pain — and both of those might be incurable. But his intake packet revealed how much his collateral damages added to his pain and complicated any efforts to treat it. Ralph began to understand that his physical suffering and dysfunction were happening in the context of what mattered to him as a unique person. So, the beginning of our work was this exploration of who he was, how much damage he had suffered, and what it meant to him.

Collecting an Existential Tool Kit

For Ralph, it was a revelation that it *mattered* what the impacts of his pain meant to him. His injuries and pain events were not just events. With a shock, he realized that no aspect of "what mattered" had been left unharmed. He had not been helped to become fully aware of this before. Nor had he understood the importance of how he reacted to his pain. Ralph began to see that he was not overreacting emotionally, being "weak," or failing to deal with the challenge of his chronic pain. But he also started to wonder if his ways of coping and getting his needs met were up to the challenges he faced.

We worked together to investigate Ralph's experience, his perception of it, and his response. From Ralph's initial resistance to change, he began to move toward being much more open to exploring how he was dealing with his challenges.

For each element of impact and response, we considered what worked for Ralph and what did not. We focused on how he usually got his needs met and how he coped with stressors. We examined his current use of coping methods to address his symptoms: All human experience translates into thoughts and feelings, which are shaped by many forces operating within us. So we worked on understanding how his method of coping determined his thoughts and feelings and how to change them to better serve outcomes of thriving.

Positive outcomes can occur through changing one's perception. Ralph achieved this by expanding his awareness of himself, his innate possibilities, and his increasing knowledge of how to get optimal performance of his existential tool kit.

Challenging Thoughts and Feelings

Ralph came to understand that his thoughts and feelings — critical tools in trying to understand his pain — were determined by his perception of his symptoms. And that, in his case, his perception had been severely limited by a lack of awareness. First, he had been unaware of the extent to which pain's impacts had damaged his life. And second, he had been unaware of the depth of his innate abilities to deal with those impacts.

This lack of awareness led his pain to produce considerably more anxiety and anger — and more stress — than necessary. Ralph was experiencing significant, continuous, severe pain any time he was awake and throughout the night. This extreme pain experience was filtered through his emotions and thoughts about it, including his lack of understanding of his diagnosis and treatment and his uncertainty about his safety from being reinjured or permanently disabled. He was addressing his pain through a coping system ill-designed to deal with this experience.

This had caused him to engage in excessive downtime and guarding and protecting behaviors. His muscles became physically de-activated and de-conditioned. He gained weight from stress eating and from lack of movement and exercise. His mental faculties, especially concentration, focus, attention, short-term memory, and decision-making, were disrupted. He lost energy and motivation, and eventually his sense of physical confidence, self-image, and identity.

Building New Ways of Coping

We next explored what had happened after Ralph's entry into treatment for his pain. It became obvious that rather than helping, in many ways his treatment was working against his recovery. He thought this must be due to a failure of the medical system or a failure on his part. Indeed, some of the setbacks were related to problems with the medical system, but many of them related to Ralph's usual ways of coping with challenges.

Because of Ralph's personal history, he found it easier to distrust than to trust his providers; he was not surprised to be disappointed or to face additional suffering when trying to get what he felt he needed. Ralph was uncomfortable talking about his feelings in general, having been raised to consider that "weak" behavior. He did not talk to anyone about how his treatment made him feel. He was not open about his emotional reaction to his pain or how his providers might help him with this. Nor did he feel comfortable being assertive about his disappointments and frustrations with his providers, for fear of being too aggressive and getting "fired" as a patient. He never shared his fears, which arose from his lack of understanding about his condition and treatment. Coping this way while being treated for persistent incurable conditions will derail successful outcomes. Unfortunately, Ralph had been unaware of this.

Ralph's approach to his providers had prevented him from learning that the first and most important concern was not pain reduction, it was understanding his pain and the treatments for it, and, most importantly, learning how to be safe from flare-ups, reinjury, or worse. To be fully engaged in his recovery, what Ralph really needed to know was how to be safe while trying to recapture as much of his physical life as he could.

These fundamental questions had yet to be answered. This made it near impossible for Ralph to proceed collaboratively and effectively through the recommended treatments.

Finally, Ralph realized that his way of coping may have served him well in the past, but now directly threatened his chances of getting his treatment needs met. Exploring this was Ralph's first introduction into the concept of optimizing the use of his existential immune system. Once he saw how his methods of coping were not adequate to the task, and what they were costing him, he was willing to change.

Partnering with Providers

So Ralph and I worked on how to prepare in advance for his meetings with his providers. We practiced communication skills to express his emotional needs as well as his physical needs. We explored proper questioning techniques for clarifying his actual diagnosis and treatment plans. Then, in his appointments, Ralph began to learn about the physical structure of his injuries and how and why they generated the pain and other symptoms they did. He learned how treatment was supposed to work, and what were realistic prognoses and expectations.

After a short time of applying these communication techniques, Ralph was feeling more certain about his physical state and the possible outcomes of treatment. More importantly, he felt much safer in his movements and less fearful of reinjury or permanent disability. He realized that pain did not always mean harm or physical threat.

The realization that much of his pain was not dangerous — just unpleasant — helped him become more physically active and also consider a more proactive approach to his physical treatment.

Following this new awareness of his physical state, Ralph and I started working on his physical re-activation and improving his physical conditioning, including through weight loss. We worked on techniques to end his sleep disruption.

After many months of effort, Ralph was feeling more empowered and in control. He reported, "I don't know if I have less pain or just don't feel the same about it." As he continued, his daily pattern of pain changed. The pain became intermittent, and he was better able to manage it when it occurred. Overall, he had less pain and less intense flare-ups. He slept more soundly and had begun to lose the excess weight. His stress over having pain was diminished. The pain had less impact on his mental faculties as well.

The change in Ralph's awareness and physical experience countered his disempowering beliefs about his pain. He felt much less helpless, hopeless, and discouraged about being able to manage or lessen his pain. He no longer experienced it as "impossible to handle or function with." He was challenging the belief that his pain was punishment or unfair. He was becoming less certain that he would be crippled or paralyzed. All these shifts helped him focus on pushing the limits of recovery.

Finally, Ralph abandoned the thought that his difficulty in handling his pain was a personal weakness. He now knew that his pain problems, while complex, were not a mystery, and that his doctors understood them.

He suspended judgment about whether his pain would be permanent or would ruin his life. He began to believe he might be able to cope with it, and possibly even go back to work again. He felt more motivated to try things, understanding that his condition would not necessarily get worse. He also realized that others might really care if he let them, and that there were many ways he could help them understand what it felt like for him.

Healing Relationships

Having focused on Ralph's physical treatment, we turned to pain's impact on his most important relationships. Prior to his injuries, Ralph had been close, loving, and engaged with his wife and his children. But Ralph's injury had changed all this. He had withdrawn emotionally and physically. He had rejected his wife's persistent offers of help, trying to pretend he was OK. When there were conflicts and communication breakdowns between them, these did not get resolved.

When I first met Ralph's wife, she was feeling completely overwhelmed, lonely, edgy, and irritable. Her sleep and all her daily routines were disrupted by caring for Ralph. She had begun to question whether she wanted to stay in the marriage, and Ralph sensed this.

Ralph had also withdrawn from his children, shutting down emotionally and refusing to do things with them because he did not want to be a "complainer." He did not explain why he was doing this, and he did not ask how they felt. In fact, Ralph was ashamed of his anxiety and anger. He was afraid the kids would think less of him if they knew how he really felt, so he stayed distant. Understandably, however, his children felt increasingly upset, distressed, and afraid. They felt that they were losing their dad altogether. Once again, Ralph's approach to coping was undermining his recovery.

Ralph had developed this style of coping in reaction to his childhood experiences. For as long as he could remember, Ralph had been pressed to take responsibility for his younger siblings. His dad had been physically abusive. His mom had been emotionally abusive. Ralph told me that he and his mom hadn't talked for years. These early experiences left Ralph with an unconscious longing to feel safe from all types of pain and to be taken care of. But, paradoxically, he had grown up to be defiant in his stance that he did not need anyone else. He entered adulthood quite cynical and having great difficulty trusting others.

When we explored Ralph's history of dealing with anxiety and anger, we discovered that he had been raised in a family environment that showed little respect for these emotions and little understanding of how to use them properly. In fact, he was punished and made to feel ashamed for having them. This left Ralph no option but to try to deny and suppress them. From being judged harshly for any behavior his caretakers did not like, Ralph learned to negatively judge himself (and others) for any similar behavior. He had been made to feel "weak" for needing to feel cared for and taken care of.

Since his injury, Ralph had experienced threats to almost all of his needs. It was no wonder he was experiencing excessive anxiety and anger—emotions he experienced as destructive to himself and to others. This left little room for compassion toward himself, or toward others when they asked for help. Whether with providers in treatment or relating to his family about his pain, this orientation toward his needs was a major hindrance to Ralph getting what he needed to recover.

> "Anxiety and anger are extremely important human emotions that have critical functioning purposes."

As Ralph came to understand the negative impacts of his childhood, he became more open to undoing the damage done. This led me to help Ralph learn that anxiety and anger are extremely important human emotions that have critical functional purposes. Anxiety is a signal that needs are being threatened and a helpful guide to finding solutions. Anger provides the focus and energy to reduce or eliminate the threats. In our work, we challenged Ralph's adherence to lessons learned about these emotions when he was young and relatively helpless. He began to see that in his life now, his lack of awareness about the importance of his emotions, and his thoughts and beliefs as well, was a bigger problem than his pain. He came to appreciate that the quality of his emotions was not the problem, nor was his thinking and beliefs—when those beliefs were based upon objective truth.

Based on Ralph's dawning awareness of his dysfunctional approaches to sharing emotion with his family, we included Ralph's wife and children in our conversations. We began by discussing the complete facts about Ralph's structural issues, his prognosis, and his treatment modalities. We addressed how these facts applied to realistic expectations about physical recovery. We moved on to sharing Ralph's new understanding about how the challenges of his personal history had created ways of coping that had inadvertently harmed his family and disempowered them. We shared alternative approaches Ralph was working on so they could join in and help him achieve significant changes in how he coped.

We worked, all together, on more effective strategies for communication and conflict resolution as well. Ralph and his family ultimately felt more grounded, informed, and empowered. They gained confidence that they knew how to master the impact that Ralph's pain had had on them. They began to rebuild their relationships and to deepen and improve them despite the suffering they had been through.

When Ralph and his family became true partners in his recovery, they were all able to reduce their stress and sense of loss.

Moving into a New Life

As Ralph and I proceeded, our focus increasingly turned to all the other impacts Ralph's pain had on him as a person. These were found in his day-to-day life, his situation, his functioning, and his experiences. They were also found in the challenges to his ways of operating as a person and the mental health issues that had been created in reaction to Ralph's pain. These included impacts on his self-image, self-efficacy, values, and identity.

Over the months we worked together, Ralph was changing. Despite his pain, he was evolving his way of operating based on a growing awareness of the obstacles his former habits raised to expressing his true self. His evolution stemmed from a focus on what was important to him and what tools he could bring to bear to help himself recover and thrive. He began to acknowledge more of how his pain had affected him as a person. He noticed how his traditional way of operating as a person was interfering with his recovery. Especially, he began to see how his old way of operating had created a disconnect from his own sense of meaning, purpose, and values.

While Ralph was exploring his existential reaction to his chronic pain and how to make constructive use of the feelings, thoughts, and beliefs it engendered, he became less depressed and less plagued by excessive anxiety, worry, anger, and frustration. He came to understand that depression was a dysfunctional way to shut down anxiety and anger. He began to see that if he started to embrace and address these feelings, it would be empowering — not self-defeating.

We also worked on other elements of his thinking process. This revealed that he held negative judgmental thoughts toward himself and others. He made excessive use of rationalizations and assumptions, and on occasion, he used magical thinking to try to manage his reaction to pain.

As Ralph began to challenge the validity of these kinds of thinking, the truth about his situation continued to become clearer to him. It became increasingly obvious that negative self-talk, unchallenged negative beliefs, and other unreliable ways of thinking were not helpful to producing an authentic and self-empowering response to his challenges. Persisting in this way of thinking had only driven him deeper into depression, self-loathing, and isolation from people who could help him. So now, rather than blame himself or others for his condition, Ralph began to have more compassion for himself and became more open to allowing others to help him.

Being Worthy of Love

Ralph's work with me, of course, took many months. Two of the biggest barriers to this part of Ralph's recovery were the uncertainty he had about his self-worth and his difficulty resolving conflicts with others. These were next to be addressed.

Ralph was quite good at giving to others, but not to himself. We began to work on his willingness to feel *equally entitled* to get what he needed. His childhood had made him question his sense of self-worth and entitlement. It had left him lacking in skills to successfully resolve conflict as well. These were major issues because he was not sure he deserved to ask for, let alone get, help. And the many stressors he dealt with bred potential for conflict every single day.

Based on Ralph's growing awareness that these dynamics were undermining his recovery, we challenged those childhood foundations. We explored why he questioned his worth and what lessons he had learned about conflict. He began to see that his beliefs about these were based on a child-like understanding of complex behavior. As a child, Ralph assumed his parents' behavior was caused by his being unworthy of love. As a child, he had understood conflict to mean that he was wrong or bad — which made conflict unresolvable.

But now Ralph could see that his parents' behavior was a reflection of their problems and limitations, not any kind of statement about him being worthy of love or conflict being unresolvable. He had the opportunity to feel worthy if he offered it to himself without conditions. And there were emotionally safe ways to resolve his differences with others. As a result, Ralph was able to feel more entitled to what he needed to help him manage his pain. He also was able to find more common ground and connection with people with whom he had differences, rather than friction and lack of resolution.

This process of Ralph evolving his operating system to cope more effectively involved a continuous building of awareness of possibilities and opportunities. It included a considerable amount of practice in the effective use of all the potential that evolution had given him. Over several years, he underwent a major personal transformation in his use of his thinking processes, beliefs, feelings, biology, and connectivity.

Ralph's growing mastery over his pain through optimal use of his existential tools resulted in many positive impacts. His marital and family stress was substantially reduced. He was able to reconnect with friends and associates in positive, meaningful ways. He was more open to people's help and emotional support. We addressed his financial worries by exploring and locating vocational options that did not depend upon a full physical recovery.

Once Ralph could acknowledge his loss of the activities he used to enjoy, he was able to retain or regain some involvement in them through careful planning and moderation. He also discovered new experiences that his pain did not interfere with — such as painting, chess, and journaling. On a daily basis he demonstrated to himself that he was far from "dysfunctional, useless, and powerless."

Now, Ralph rarely feels stuck down in the dumps. He feels less sadness or discouragement — it's even possible for him to feel happy on occasion. Overall, he feels much less anxious and worried, restless and jumpy. His life feels much safer. Gone is the everyday frustration, upset, irritability, and anger he used to experience. He now experiences his pain and limitations as positive challenges that lead him to find out how he can counter them. And Ralph's self-esteem has lifted as he learned to appreciate how hard he works to overcome his challenges. Best, Ralph now values himself for who he truly is.

VAL'S STORY: SAME AND DIFFERENT

Ralph's story is not an extreme, but is in fact typical for the clients I work with. The basic process of revealing negative realities and optimizing the existential immune system is the same with all my clients, no matter how that manifests in each case and what is needed for mastery. What's different between clients is the overall level of impact on their functioning, their current resources and supports, and the current level of optimization of their existential immune system.

As you can see from reading Ralph's story, the process of working toward mastery can be quite complex. Assessing the impacts of chronic pain and educating yourself about the extent and detail of your reality is the first challenge. Exploring who you are and how you operate can also be daunting and difficult. The task of learning the techniques described in this book, at whatever level they are needed, depends in large measure on the level of commitment you are willing to make. It requires a commitment to seeking possibilities and opportunities and a willingness to change, no matter how anxiety-producing or painful the process.

While Ralph's story is representative of the stories I often encounter with new clients, each person is a unique individual, including in where they start from physically and emotionally and in their openness to personal growth. So what is the same about each person with chronic pain? *We all start out with issues with how we use our thoughts and feelings, underlying questions about self-worth, and a sense that we cannot hope to master our pain.* While the principles of mastery apply in all cases, they must be tailored to each unique individual's current existential state. Val's story demonstrates a different manifestation from Ralph's and illustrates just how adaptable the approach used in this book is.

I could share many more stories from the hundreds of clients I have worked with, but instead I'd like to use just one story — Val's story — to highlight what is the same and what is different across all my clients and, I believe, everyone living with chronic pain. I hope this will illustrate the power of the existential immune system to help you master your chronic pain.

> "Chronic pain can expose long-held secrets—and paths forward."

Optimizing One's Existential Skills

Val was an extraordinarily successful businesswoman — intelligent, skilled, and insightful. When we met, she appeared to be a highly evolved and aware person. She had been in psychological treatment and other self-discovery activities for most of her life. She was truly inspired in her work. Despite this, she had chronic pain in her hip and lower back that she just could not resolve. She believed that her current way of coping should be sufficient to deal with the challenges of her pain. Unfortunately, she was quite unaware of the existential challenges it presented her.

Val was used to being in charge. She was at a high level of management and accustomed to feeling in control. Since childhood, she had developed a nearly airtight presentation of herself. However, her advanced level of awareness and knowledge of herself did not extend to her reactions to the fears and negative lessons learned in her early childhood. These were deeply repressed and suppressed. She kept her negative feelings to herself and was heavily inclined to use negative self-talk and rationalization as a way of motivating herself. She had yet to fully integrate her thinking and emotions for optimal performance. In other words, her existential immune system was compromised.

Despite Val's best defenses, her unresolved early emotional experiences and subsequent dysfunctions in her thinking and feeling were being reactivated by her chronic pain. Yet Val was unaware of all of this. She couldn't understand how her dysfunctional use of her feelings and thoughts was undermining her. She did not realize that her way of operating reflected one priority: that she never appear to be vulnerable or feel a lack of control. Her way of operating and coping could not handle being put in a dependent position.

Thus her chronic pain exposed her long-held secret.

At first I was awed by her insight and self-awareness, and confused by her reaction to pain. Her psychological defenses were so flawless, I could hardly see past them. Her hidden issues were revealed through the unraveling of the "mystery" of her limited physical recovery. Like in a detective novel, there were clues that pointed to the source of her difficulty. The first clue was that she engaged in an excessive amount of negative self-judgment and was unaware of it. In addition, she had been in several unsuccessful marriages and relationships — despite her superior communication skills. And even though she had been highly successful and respected in the business world, she felt somehow "unsatisfied and unfulfilled."

Building Self-Worth

When we explored Val's family history, we discovered the source of her problems in managing her pain. She had grown up in a demanding environment, one that determined for her who she should be and what she should do with her life. She was never given a choice about what she wanted. At the same time, she was raised to believe that if she needed to complain about anything, there was something wrong with *her*. This upbringing, no matter how well intentioned, had ended up inhibiting her ability to engage proactively with her family, providers, and friends to get her needs met when facing challenges. Our conversations about this revealed an underlying lack of self-worth and scant sense of entitlement. Val had done a good job of covering up her fears, but dealing with her feelings of helplessness due to her chronic pain was challenging her sense of worth.

Committing to Change

At that point, each session became a challenge in which Val tried to convince me she did not need help. As a counter, I demonstrated all the different ways in which she was not able to help herself. It was hard for Val to recognize this, but eventually she was able to acknowledge the need

> "When you succeed in connecting to vulnerability, new possibilities open."

to evolve her operating system. This was the real beginning of our work together. Eventually, Val was able to embrace feeling safe, secure, and good about herself without always having to be in control, in charge, and invulnerable. Emotionally, her new connection to her own vulnerability allowed her to better process her reactions to the impacts of her pain and opened possibilities that she could not have accessed before.

Over time, Val began to see the continuing need to upgrade her operating system so she could get what she needed more effectively, especially from others. She already had the inspiration in her own life to do her work, but she wasn't yet able to easily tap into the inspiration of others in her life to help her. Opening up this potential eventually not only led to reconciling her childhood issues, but created a true sense of family and community for the first time in her life. Bringing together the forces of her own personal inspiration and that of others greatly increased her ability to master her chronic pain. The result: Val's pain ceased to be the centerpiece in her life.

COMMON GROUND IN CHRONIC PAIN

Ralph and Val are just two of the multitude of clients I have worked with. I believe their stories illustrate what can be accomplished. What all my clients have in common is that they are suffering from the impacts of chronic pain and need a more effective way to deal with and master it.

In my practice, I work with clients of all ages and many individual differences. They come from many walks of life, vocations, and life situations. They are single, married, with or without children. They have experienced enormous success and life satisfaction, complete absence of either, and everything in between. They represent the gamut of personality and coping types, life configurations, and levels of mental health or emotional problems. They arrive at varying levels of dysfunction. Every person is unique. Everyone requires an approach that is customized to meet their uniqueness.

Every person's suffering begin as a mystery: Who is this person? How do they operate to get their needs met? Why is this approach a problem for them? There are no wrong ways to start. My clients are not broken or defective. Each person has their own approach to operating in the world—just as you do. But many ways of operating come with side effects, and sometimes those side effects are significant enough to overcome any benefit. This work takes time, patience, and perseverance from my clients and myself. In all cases, respect and trust between my client and myself must come first.

IN CONCLUSION

By now, you've developed a much deeper understanding of just how complicated chronic pain really is. This knowledge may already have helped you become aware of the extent of the impacts your pain has caused you. It's likely you've begun to learn how to use your own existential immune system to help with these impacts. It may be a long journey, but I hope I have demonstrated that it is a journey worth taking.

I understand how hard it is to believe it's possible to truly make the changes this book suggests. I understand that you've been faced with many challenges already. It may be daunting to embrace faith and hope and a willingness to try again. When I started working in pain management, I asked myself, "Can I really hope to help people who are suffering this much?" Thankfully, the answer is yes!

What continues to motivate me to write and speak about this journey are the clients who have come to me willing to seek inspiration and tap into their potential to master their chronic pain. I want others who are unaware of what can be done to see: *This is possible*. Life is full of existential challenges; chronic pain is only one of many. To be human is to be vulnerable. To be human is also to be born with the potential to deal with that ability. Repeatedly, in the years that I have worked in this field, I have seen people experience incredible challenges — physical, emotional, psychological, existential. And I have seen these people find ways to find inspiration, to evolve, to transform, to change, to regain their lives and thrive. They have been good teachers for me. And it is for them — and for everyone else who can benefit from their examples — that this book is written.

By making use of everything in this book, working with help and guidance and constant awareness, practice, and commitment, you *can* master chronic pain. Does this mean you will no longer have any physical pain or life impact? Every situation is different. What I do know is that the people who go through this process become considerably more functional and more in charge of their lives. They rediscover themselves. They find a way to thrive despite any remaining pain, and to live with considerably less physical, emotional, psychological, and existential impact. So, I invite you to take the next step to begin your evolution to mastery.

Tools

The self-evaluation forms in these appendixes were developed to help you assess how you have been impacted by chronic pain:

- Appendix A corresponds to part 2, "The Physical Experience."
- Appendix B corresponds to part 3, "The Personal Experience."
- Appendix C corresponds to part 4, "The Treatment Experience."

You can use these forms whenever you like: before you read each section; after you read the whole book; or repeatedly, to track how your experience changes over time.

It may be useful to complete each set of forms before you read the corresponding chapters. This can help you recognize which ones will be the most relevant and useful to your particular experience. In my practice, I have new clients complete the forms before our first session together. They report finding this exercise educational, informative, and even enlightening, and I hope this will be the case for you as well. Additional forms are available on the New Options website.

Appendixes

Self-Evaluation Forms

Appendix A
Physical Impact Assessments

A-1. Physical Impacts Inventory

Read each statement. Check (√) the column that indicates how true you believe that statement to be TODAY. Please address all the items.

My experience today is that …	0—Not at all	1—Somewhat	2—Moderately	3—A lot	4—Extremely
Sleep Disruption					
I sleep lightly or wake easily in the night					
I cannot fall asleep easily					
I wake many times during the night					
When I wake, I stay awake for long periods without being able to fall back asleep					
I wake up earlier than planned					
I do not feel rested or restored after sleep					
I sleep excessively					
Physical De-activation					
I engage in avoidance behaviors (e.g., thoughts, feelings, behaviors, and experiences; avoiding daily responsibilities; sleeping excessively; using substances)					
I cannot engage in ordinary movement (e.g., walking, sitting up, lifting)					
I cannot complete important tasks (e.g., household, work, recreational, relationship, family)					
I engage in guarding and protecting behaviors (e.g., avoiding certain movements, trying not to bend or kneel, sitting sideways to dress, lifting with only one side)					
I engage in excessive downtime (e.g., sitting, lying down, being inactive)					
I cannot engage in daily routines					
I cannot engage in daily activities					
I cannot complete activities of daily living (e.g., bathing, brushing teeth, dressing)					
I cannot use proper body mechanics					
I use a prosthetic device (e.g., cane, back brace, walker, crutches)					

Physical De-conditioning					
I have a restricted range of motion					
I have medical complications					
I have damage to physical systems (e.g., immune system, breathing, circulation)					
I've gained or lost weight					
My pain tolerance has decreased					
I've lost strength					
I've lost flexibility					
I've lost function (e.g., ability to do or complete physical tasks or be physically independent)					
I've lost physical comfort					
Physical tension in my body has increased					
I have impaired motor control					
I have poor balance					
I have decreased mobility					
I have more medical problems					
I have more complications to existing medical conditions					
I have physical atrophy					
I have little energy					
Cognitive Impact					
I have poor attention					
I have poor concentration					
I have poor short-term memory					
I have poor mental flexibility					
I have poor verbal ability					
I have poor mental processing (speed and response)					
I have difficulty completing tasks					
I have poor motor performance					
I have poor executive function (e.g., ability to use memory, concentration, attention, focus, and problem-solving to monitor, manage, and achieve goals)					
I have poor multitasking ability					
I have poor reaction time					
I have poor decision-making ability					
I have poor long-term memory					

A-2. Post-Injury Physical Experience Inventory

Read each statement. Check (√) the column that indicates how true you believe that statement to be SINCE YOUR INJURY OR ILLNESS. Please address all the items.

Since my injury or illness ...	0—Not at all	1—Somewhat	2—Moderately	3—A lot	4—Extremely
I've reduced or discontinued my activities					
I spend a lot of time each day sitting or lying down					
I don't do a lot of tasks I used to do					
I've lost physical conditioning					
I use my body differently in order to avoid pain					
I've gained weight					
I have a lower pain tolerance					
My muscles are weaker					
I'm less flexible					
I have less energy					
My sleep is disturbed					
I feel more physically vulnerable					
I've lost physical confidence					
I've lost valued roles					
My self-image is diminished					
My physical identity has been lost					
I feel less confident					
I feel less capable					
I feel less competent					
I've lost physical comfort					
I feel less safe and secure					
I've become more dependent on others					
I've become more fearful of mortality					
I find dealing with my pain to be physically draining					
I feel diminished in others' eyes					

A-3. Emotional and Psychological Impacts Inventory

Read each statement. Check (√) the column that indicates how true you believe that statement to be OVERALL. Please address all the items.

My experience overall is that ...	0—Not at all	1—Somewhat	2—Moderately	3—A lot	4—Extremely
I've lost physical identity					
I've lost self-image					
I've lost self-worth					
I've lost self-confidence					
I've lost self-acceptance					
I've lost social acceptance and inclusion					
I think others have negative perceptions of me					
I have more self-doubt					
I see myself as disabled					
I see myself as a patient or a diagnosis, not a person					
I've lost a sense of belonging					
I have a negative body image					
I feel marginalized					
I feel discriminated against					
I avoid difficult challenges					
I cannot engage in daily activities					
I cannot complete activities of daily living (e.g., bathing, brushing teeth, dressing)					
I cannot use proper body mechanics					
I use a prosthetic device (e.g., cane, back brace, walker, crutches)					

A-4. Physical Impacts Checklist

Read each statement. Check (√) all items that apply to your pain experience.

√	
	I experience significant pain (many hours per day)
	I experience pain at all times of day
	I experience pain in multiple physical areas of my body
	I experience pain at a disturbing and concerning level (6–10 on a scale of 0–10)
	Pain has significantly affected my ability to get things done
	Pain has caused significant sleep disruption (multiple awakenings related to pain, non-restful and fitful sleep)
	Certain activities immediately causes pain (bending, lifting, coughing, sneezing)
	I experience pain at a moderate to more severe level
	My condition is worse now than at the time of my original treatment
	My condition is worsening over time
	I have no positive expectations for pain reductions in the future
	I spend an excessive amount of time sitting or lying down
	I change my position frequently
	I avoid doing household chores
	I have difficulty dressing
	I use handrails and other supports when moving around
	My pain interferes with activities
	I walk more slowly
	I find it difficult to stand up
	I get dressed more slowly
	I am aware of pain during the majority of the day and night
	Guarding and protecting behaviors – (avoids certain movements, tries not to bend or kneel, lies sideways in bed, sits sideways to dress, lifts with the left side)
	I've lost the ability to do certain activities
	I've lost the ability to do certain tasks
	I'm unable to do my favorite tasks or activities
	I use a potentially addictive medication
	My medications cause side effects that undermine functioning

	I've lost physical conditioning
	I've lost athleticism
	This is my first physical injury
	I am physically weaker, with less flexible muscles and less energy
	I've gained weight
	I have new physical problems related to my medications
	I've lost physical identity
	I've lost physical competence
	I've lost physical confidence
	I am more physically dependent on others
	I've lost physical self-image
	I've lost physical strength and confidence
	I feel unrelenting pain and discomfort
	My pain is unpredictable, with no patterns or control of flare-ups
	I am dependent on medication

Personal Impacts
Assessments

B-1. Personal Experience Inventory

Read each statement. Check (√) the column that indicates how true you believe that statement to be SINCE YOUR INJURY OR ILLNESS. Please address all the items.

The pain from my injury or illness has ...	0—Not at all	1—Somewhat	2—Moderately	3—A lot	4—Extremely
Impacted my lifestyle					
Reduced my pleasure and/or satisfaction in life					
Limited my opportunities					
Changed my social and economic status					
Changed my expectations					
Undermined my capacity to enjoy life					
Changed my pursuits					
Led to the loss of satisfying social activities					
Undermined my ability to take good care of myself					
Undermined my sense of well-being					
Interfered with me learning new things					
Interfered with me having new and satisfying experiences					
Reduced my ability to feel productive					
Limited my potential or ability to sustain effort					
Affected my memory, concentration, attention, and/or focus					
Led to loss of relationships					
Made me feel alienated from others					
Damaged my relationships					
Undermined my ability to cope					
Made me feel insecure					
Made me feel ashamed of myself					
Made it hard for me to be the person I want to be					
Made me less confident					

	0	1	2	3	4
Made me less competent					
Caused emotional or psychological problems					
Made me feel like I'm not myself					
Gotten in the way of the way I want my life to be					
Made me lose or change roles					
Made me feel too dependent on others					
Made me develop negative beliefs about pain					
Made me fearful of pain					
Made me fearful of engaging in most activity of any kind					
Made me fearful of re-injuring myself					
Made me fearful of rehabilitation					
Convinced me I'm disabled					
Made me preoccupied with my pain					
Made me fearful of mortality					

B-2. Personal Impacts Checklist

Read each statement. Check (√) all items that apply to your pain experience.

	PERSONAL MEANING Since my injury or illness ...
	I've experienced major impacts to my life
	I've experienced breakdowns in coping abilities
	I've experienced loss of personal style
	I've experienced loss of self-efficacy
	I've experienced dysfunctional, negative thoughts or self-talk
	I've had repeated thoughts of past negative experiences that involved feeling victimized and helpless
	I've developed a pain phobia
	I've felt that my failure to recover is a personal failure
	I've had repeated thoughts of past trauma
	I've had repeated thoughts of past injury or pain
	I've felt diminished as a person
	I've felt that I'm paying for life with pain
	I have fear of the future
	PERSONAL IDENTITY Since my injury or illness ...
	I've felt disconnected from my sense of a past or future self
	I've experienced loss of autonomy
	I've failed to fulfill important roles, such as spouse, parent, provider, friend, or worker
	I've experienced relationship instability
	I've experienced dysfunctional beliefs
	I've experienced motional instability
	I've experienced breakdowns in problem-solving abilities
	I've experienced breakdowns in following or succeeding with treatment
	I've experienced chronic stress
	I've developed negative pain beliefs

	PERSONAL DEVELOPMENT During my childhood ...
	I did not feel taken care of
	I experienced abuse/neglect
	I did not feel privileged
	I experienced emotional enmeshment (e.g., unclear personal boundaries between myself and others)
	I experienced childhood trauma
	I experienced parental injury, illness, unhappiness
	I experienced family instability
	I was expected to play a parental role

B-3. Risk Factors for Injury Inventory

Read each statement. Check (√) the column that indicates how true you believe that statement to be ABOUT YOUR CHILDHOOD AND LIFE EXPERIENCES. Please address all the items.

During my childhood ...	0—Not at all	1—Somewhat	2—Moderately	3—A lot	4—Extremely
I experienced abandonment by a parent or other significant family member					
My parents divorced					
One or both of my parents was harsh, punitive, distant, or cold					
I experienced physical abuse					
I experienced sexual abuse					
I experienced emotional abuse					
I experienced neglect					
I experienced trauma					
I was expected to play a "parent" role					
There was a lot of interpersonal conflict in the household					
I experienced significant loss					
One or both of my parents engaged in substance abuse					
One or both of my parents suffered from chronic illness or injury					
I suffered from chronic illness or injury					
I experienced special value for being sick					
One or both of my parents paid excessive attention to or worried over physical problems					
A member of my household was disabled					
A member of my household was unable to leave the house					
The time my chronic pain began was the first time I was injured					
There seemed to be no relationship between my pain and my diagnosed injury					

	0	1	2	3	4
I was diagnosed with depression					
I was diagnosed with hypochondria					
I was diagnosed with an anxiety disorder					
I was diagnosed with schizophrenia					
I was diagnosed with a dissociative disorder					
I repressed my emotions					
I saw myself as a victim					
I had problems trusting people					
I had a very limited social life					
I placed a great deal of value on self-sacrifice					

B-4. Social-Emotional Impacts Checklist

Read each statement. Check (√) all items that apply to your pain experience.

√	
	I feel traumatized by my pain
	I've lost connections, relationships, and social activities with friends and family
	I lack exercise
	I experience social isolation
	I worry over my health
	I'm uncertain about how much I can recover
	I'm uncertain about how safe I am physically
	I experience anxiety
	I experience anger
	I experience depression
	I experience excessive worry or frustration
	I experience significant loss of motivation
	I experience increased dependence
	I experience increased vulnerability
	I experience increased fear of mortality
	I have become cynical, judgmental, or mistrusting
	Reduced pleasure and satisfaction in life
	Changed expectations
	I've lost opportunities
	I've lost pleasurable pursuits
	My socioeconomic status has changed
	Undermined self-care and self-image
	I've lost my sense of well-being
	Challenge to the possibility of success
	I've lost important roles
	I feel unhappy
	I feel unsatisfied
	I feel unproductive
	I feel unrewarded
	I feel unaccomplished

	I've lost a sense of fun
	I've lost a sense of playfulness
	I've lost a sense of joy
	I've lost a sense of safety and security
	I've lost a sense of hope and optimism
	I've lost a sense of self-efficacy
	Failure of coping system lost stoicism, keeping negative feelings to self,
	I've lost a sense of being independent
	I've lost a sense of patience
	I've lost a sense of peace
	I've lost a sense of spirituality
	I've lost a sense of autonomy
	I've lost the feeling of being worthwhile, respectable, or likable
	I feel guilt and shame
	I blame myself
	I feel a sense of alienation
	I'm afraid of pain
	I'm afraid of pain permanence
	I'm afraid injuring myself again
	I'm afraid of flare-ups of pain or injury
	I'm afraid of activity
	I'm afraid of disability
	I'm afraid of mortality
	I'm afraid of being weak
	I'm afraid of being disabled
	I feel fragile
	I'm afraid my treatment outcomes will be limited and not complete
	I'm afraid my pain will cause excessive functional impact
	I'm afraid my pain will never stop
	I experience fears of the future
	I have post-traumatic stress disorder

Appendix C

Treatment Experience Assessments

C-1. Treatment Confusion Inventory

Read each statement. Check (√) the column that indicates how true you believe that statement to be TODAY. Please address all the items.

My experience today is that ...	0—Not at all	1—Somewhat	2—Moderately	3—A lot	4—Extremely
I'm confused about my actual diagnosis—it's ambiguous, indefinite, confusing, and/or contradictory					
My treatment has failed, and I don't really understand why					
My expectations about getting a clear diagnosis have been disappointed					
My treatment has not been managed, coordinated, or integrated					
I've been sent from specialist to specialist in a manner that doesn't improve my condition and adds to my confusion					
I've been damaged further by my treatment					
My treatment experience has made me fearful of treatment					
My treatment has created a dependence on medication					
I'm tired of treatment					
I don't know why I'm in pain					
I don't know what my treatments are for or why					
I don't know which treatment works or doesn't work					
I don't have a coherent, comprehensive, and integrated plan of treatment					
I don't know who is in charge of my treatment					
I don't know if all my providers are on the same team					
I don't know why my providers can't seem to diagnose my condition					
I don't know why my providers can't come up with a treatment that works					
I don't know what it means when my treatment doesn't work					

	0	1	2	3	4
I don't know why my providers can't tell me what's going to happen					
I don't know if I've found the right provider					
I don't know how much of my life history my providers need to know to understand my needs					

C-2. Treatment Experience Inventory

Read each statement. Check (√) the column that indicates how true you believe that statement to be SINCE YOUR ILLNESS OR INJURY. Please address all the items.

Since my injury or illness, my experience is that ...	0—Not at all	1—Somewhat	2—Moderately	3—A lot	4—Extremely
My providers and I really understand each other					
I believe my providers and I are in this together					
I believe my providers and I communicate really well					
I know what my role is in my treatment					
I know what questions to ask my providers					
I know how much of my needs I should talk about with my providers					
My providers and I have shared concepts about my problem					
My providers and I have a strong partnership					
My providers and I are fully prepared for our encounters					
My providers and I clearly and completely express our needs					
My providers and I express both positive and negative reactions to our encounters					
I clearly understand both my role as a patient and my providers' role in my treatment					
My providers share with me all the important and crucial information about my condition					
I share with my providers all the important and crucial information about my condition					
My providers ask me all their most important questions, and I answer					
I ask my providers all my most important questions, and they answer					
My providers clearly diagnose my condition in a way I understand					
My providers offer concrete, positive, understandable treatment plans					

	0	1	2	3	4
My providers meet my treatment needs					
My providers communicate well					
My providers educate me about my condition					
My providers tell me what to do to help my condition in a comprehensive and understandable fashion					
My providers understand my suffering and my need for relief					
My providers make me feel well cared for					

Which of your individual providers would score high on this scale?

_____

_____

_____

_____

_____

_____

_____

_____

_____

_____

_____

_____

_____

_____

_____

C-3. Treatment Visit Evaluation Inventory

Read each statement. Check (√) the column that indicates how true you believe that statement to be AT YOUR MOST RECENT MEDICAL APPOINTMENT. Please address all the items.

At my last appointment, my experience is that ...	0—Not at all	1—Somewhat	2—Moderately	3—A lot	4—Extremely
I had enough time at my appointment to get what I needed					
I never felt rushed					
I felt I had my provider's full attention					
I felt my provider was sufficiently knowledgeable about my condition					
I felt my provider was respectful					
I felt my provider carefully listened to me and my concerns					
My provider demonstrated as much concern for how I feel about my condition as they did about my physical condition					
My provider asked enough questions to ascertain how my physical condition is affecting my life					
My provider gave me enough information about my condition, treatments, studies, referrals, and expectations					

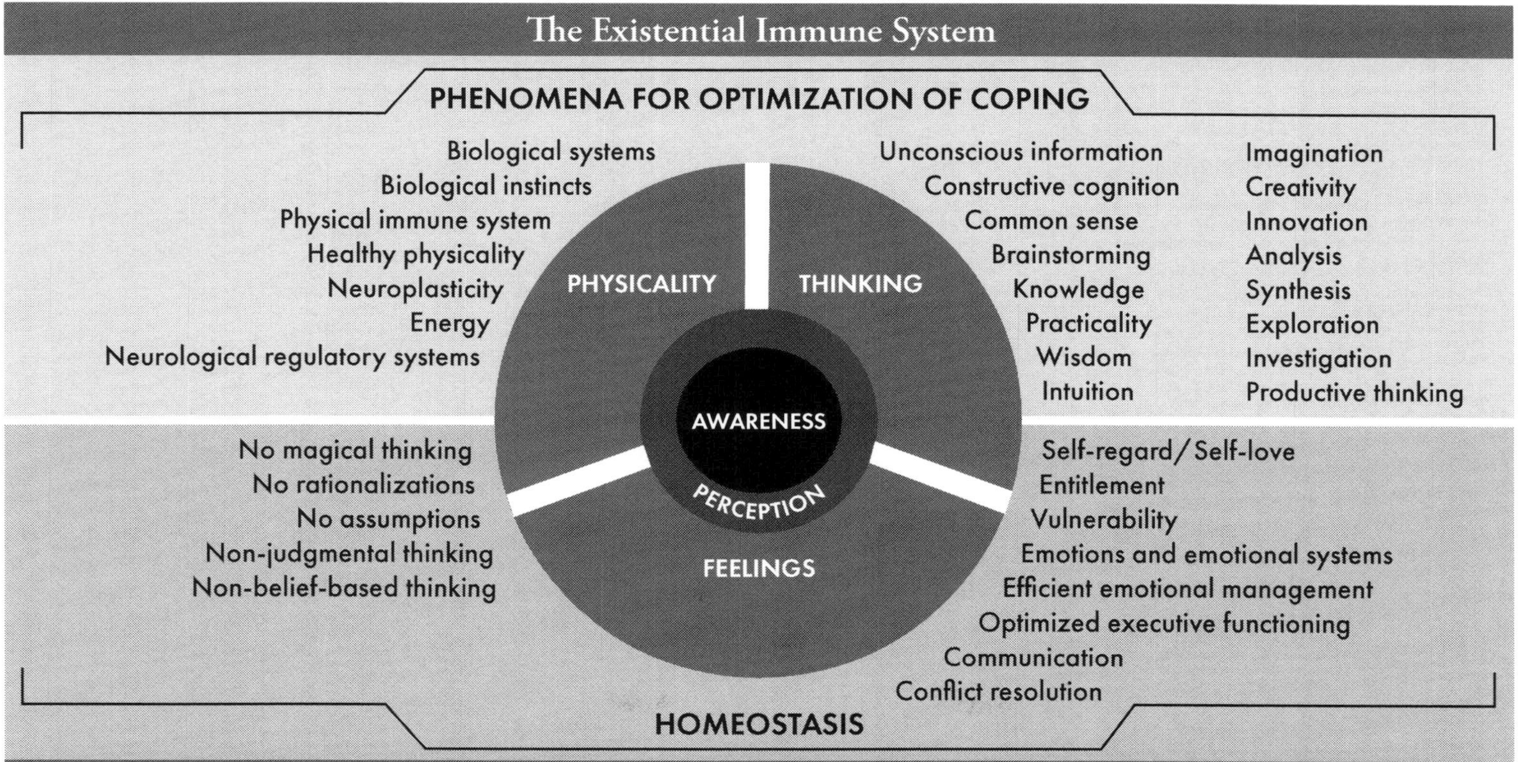

The Existential Immune System

PHENOMENA FOR OPTIMIZATION OF COPING

THINKING

Imagination
Creativity
Innovation
Analysis
Synthesis
Exploration
Investigation
Productive thinking

Unconscious information
Constructive cognition
Common sense
Brainstorming
Knowledge
Practicality
Wisdom
Intuition

No magical thinking
No rationalizations
No assumptions
Non-judgmental thinking
Non-belief-based thinking

PHYSICALITY

Biological systems
Biological instincts
Physical immune system
Healthy physicality
Neuroplasticity
Energy
Neurological regulatory systems

AWARENESS

PERCEPTION

FEELINGS

Self-regard/Self-love
Entitlement
Vulnerability
Emotions and emotional systems
Efficient emotional management
Optimized executive functioning
Communication
Conflict resolution

HOMEOSTASIS

Figure 1. Like our physical immune system, our "existential immune system" is adaptive and protective, warding off that which threatens to do harm to our non-corporeal aspects — our cognitive, emotional, perceptive, and spiritual selves. And like with the physical immune system, there are ways to optimize its functioning: through practicing awareness; making conscious choices; and cultivating compassionate, assertive, discerning self-care.

Index

About the Author

At twelve years old, after nearly dying in a diving accident, young Alan Weisser developed an unshakable belief that he could and would recover. But over a two-year physical recovery, he came to understand that it was not just physical pain that affected him. The injury had also caused a high level of emotional suffering, and severely shaken his self-confidence.

The insights from this seminal experience would emerge again later to inform his life as a clinician, but first he spent several years trying to regain his risk-taking, growth-oriented self, including becoming a trial lawyer, taking up martial arts (which became a lifelong study), and traveling. In Marrakesh, Morocco, continuing to seek what was truly important and inspiring to him, his curiosity led him to embrace the simpler life available there, where he lived for several months in organic relationship with himself, others, and his environment. He spent a great deal of time in community with a nomadic tribe and in friendship with the shaman of the tribe, gaining insights about life through lessons that mirrored his immersion in the martial arts. Coming to feel truly grounded in who he was and what inspired him, he decided it was time to return home and pursue a career in clinical psychology.

Through New Options, his group practice in pain management, Dr. Weisser has participated in multidisciplinary teams that have forged successful collaborations between clients; claim managers; physicians and medical practices; rehabilitation specialists; agencies such as the University of Washington Department of Rehabilitation; Seattle Spine & Sports Medicine; Puget Sound Sports & Spine Physicians (now at Harborview Medical Center); and other community resources. He has presented on the New Options approach in caring for people with complex and chronic pain to physicians at UW, Labor & Industries (Washington State), the National Assoc. of Spine Specialists, the Defense Trial Lawyers Assoc., and numerous medical and rehabilitation practices. By focusing on collaborative and realistic goals and practices within a coherent clinical model, Dr. Weisser's practice continues to empower people with chronic pain to transition from dysfunction and disability to empowerment and recovery.

Dr. Weisser lives in the Seattle area with his wife, Sondra, and their cat, Mr. Bubbles. Surrounded by a beautiful garden, by a bay overlooking the Olympic mountains and western sunsets, he continues to practice martial arts, work with patients, write books, develop his artwork and poetry, and follow a lifelong ambition to play lead guitar.